GOLDBERG'S
DIET
CATALOG

Also by Larry Goldberg

Goldberg's Pizza Book

GOLDBERG'S DIET CATALOG

Larry Goldberg

COLLIER BOOKS

A Division of Macmillan Publishing Co., Inc.

New York

COLLIER MACMILLAN PUBLISHERS

London

Macmillan Publishing Co., Inc.
866 Third Avenue, New York, N.Y. 10022
Collier Macmillan Canada, Ltd.

"Sandwich" (sculpture) on p. xvii by Oliver Johnston.
"Coca Cola" (lithograph) on p. xviii by Jan Cremer, 1969. Collection of
Chermayeff & Geismar Associates Inc.
Cartoons on pp. xxv and 66 from the book HAPPINESS IS A SAD SONG by
Charles M. Schulz.
Copyright © 1967 United Feature Syndicate, Inc.
Drawing on p. 1 by Paul Davis.
Drawing on p. 33 by Koren; © 1975 The New Yorker Magazine, Inc.
Cartoon on p. 97 by Vincent R. Marchica.
Cartoon on p. 114 by Ward.
Cartoon on pp. 147–151 by Wallop Manyum.
Drawing on p. 162 by Koren; © 1974 The New Yorker Magazine, Inc.
Drawing on p. 165 by Don Freeman, courtesy of the Margo Feiden Galleries, New
York City.
Drawing on p. 168 by Sasha Chermayeff.

"The Ordeal of Fats Goldberg," copyright © 1971 by Calvin Trillin, first
appeared in *The New Yorker* and published in *American Fried* by Calvin Trillin.
Reprinted by permission of Doubleday & Company, Inc.

The Introduction first appeared in the December 30, 1973 issue of the *Chicago
Tribune* Magazine under the title of "Fat Larry's Diet Resolution."

Library of Congress Cataloging in Publication Data
Goldberg, Larry.
  Goldberg's diet catalog.
    1. Obesity—United States—Societies, etc.—
Directories.   2. Reducing—United States—Societies,
etc.—Directories.   3. Reducing diets—Bibliography.
4. Food, Dietetic—Catalogs.   5. Reducing—
Equipment and supplies—Catalogs.   I. Title.
II. Title: Diet catalog.
RC628.G67   1977   613.2′5′02573   77-24898
ISBN 0-02-544480-8
ISBN 0-02-059000-8 pbk.

Design and layout: Robert Bull/Craven & Evans
First Collier Books Edition 1977

Goldberg's Diet Catalog is also published in a hardcover edition by Macmillan
Publishing Co., Inc.

Printed in the United States of America

DEDICATION

To all that made this book both possible and necessary.

Kansas City: The Bosom and Kitchen of Ma Goldberg; the Grocery Store of Pa Goldberg; the Peanut Butter of my sister, Joc; Winstead's cheeseburgers; Dolly Madison Cake Co.; Arthur Bryant Bar B Que; Zarda Dairy banana splits; Putsch's Coffee House French toast; Kresge chili dogs; LaMar's Do-Nuts; Topsy's popcorn and caramel corn; the cafeterias of Central Junior High School (cherry cobbler), Paseo High School (mashed potatoes and spaghetti), and K.C. Junior College (ham salad sandwiches); Meal-A-Minute (gone); Brownies Cafe chili burgers (gone); Big Six hamburgers (gone); Kreamy Kap Root Beer Stand (gone); Rosedale Bar B Que; R.C.'s Lounge (fried chicken and gravy); Blues Baseball Stadium Hot Dogs (great mustard); Golden Ox steaks; McLain Bakery; Ranch House griddle cakes (gone); Woolworth's hot beef sandwiches; Country Club Dairy milkshakes (gone); various bar mitzvahs; Forum Cafeteria; Roy and Ray's Drive-In; Camp Osceola Boy Scout Camp mess hall (chipped beef on toast, belly wash, vanilla pudding); front and back seat of my '37 Oldsmobile (my rolling dining rooms).

University of Missouri at Columbia, Missouri: Zeta Beta Tau Fraternity kitchen; Zana Mae Smith and Mitchell Eaton, cooks; Tastee Freeze (gone); Clark's Soda Luncheonette; Central Dairy chocolate milk; Broadway Donut Shop; M. Bar, Italian Village; Ernie's (banana cream pie); Crown Drug Store (grilled cheese sandwiches); refreshment stands at the Hall, Tiger, Missouri, and Varsity movie theaters; donuts at the AE Phi Sorority House after football games; The Pizza House; Campus Grocery Store; composing room of Columbia *Missourian;* Minute Inn; The Shack's hamburgers; The Bengal Shop; The Stables (greasy burgers).

Chicago: The refrigerator of Mr. and Mrs. Leonard Schram; Uno Pizzeria; Pick and Take in lobby of *Chicago Tribune* Tower; B & G Coffee Shop (scrambled eggs); The Squirrel Cage (gone); Demars Coffee Shop; Siegel's Delicatessen (hard salami sandwiches); Forum Cafeteria (when I had money); Aunt Susie's Restaurant (pancakes); No-Man's Land Ice Cream Stand (gone); Hackney's hamburgers and onion rings; Sara Lee cakes discount store; The Tavern Club; Ashkenaz Delicatessen; Villa Girgenti (pizza); McDonalds; Palmer House (fried perch on Fridays); Wrigley Field.

New York: The Gaiety delicatessens; The Palm and Palm Too restaurants; Nathans (french fries); Sweets Fish Restaurant; Salnet Grocery Store; Green Derby (hamburgers); Bagel Nosh; Trattoria Alfredo (Fettucini Alfredo); Entenmann's Walnut Danish Ring; Juniors Delicatessen; P. J. Berenstein Delicatessen; Four 'N 20 Pies (dutch apple); Zabars (smoked turkey); ice cream stand in Lincoln Center (summertime only); Coach House (corn sticks and chocolate cake); McDonalds; Executive Dining Room *New York Daily News;* Yankee Stadium and Shea Stadium.

CONTENTS

PREFACE

My friend Larry Goldberg, the pizza baron, is slim, but I still think of him as Fats Goldberg. So does he. Although he has "been down," as he puts it, for eighteen years, after twenty-five years of exceptional fatness, he sees himself not as a man who weighs one hundred and sixty but as a man who is constantly in danger of weighing three hundred and twenty. "Inside, I'm still a fat man," he sometimes says. When Fats and I were boys in Kansas City, he was already renowned for his corpulence—though I can't say I was ever approached about posing for Refugee Relief ads in those days myself. During college, at the University of Missouri, he reached three hundred pounds and became known as both Fats Goldberg and Three Cases Goldberg—Columbia, Missouri, having been, through a derivation process that must still puzzle students of the language, the only place in the country where anybody recognized a one-hundred-pound unit of measurement called the case. I occasionally saw him when I visited Columbia, where he was one of a number of storied eaters. According to one tale, when a restaurant near the campus instituted a policy of giving customers all they wanted to eat on Sunday nights for a dollar thirty-five, a fraternity brother of Fats's called Hog Silverman, who weighed less than two and a half cases, went over one Sunday and put it out of business. Fats was known not only for that kind of single-sitting tour de force but for the fact that he never stopped eating. When he talks about those days, a lot of his sentences begin with phrases like "Then on the way to lunch I'd stop off at the Tastee-Freez . . ."

Although Fats has never cared much for salad, he used to eat just about anything else within reach. He had a catholicity of taste comparable to that of a southern eater I once heard mentioned as being happy to eat "just about everything except Coke bottles." His specialty, though, was always junk food. "I did not get fat on *coq au vin*," he once told me. Candy bars. Lunch-meat sandwiches on white bread. Sweet rolls. Hamburgers. Chili dogs. Cake. Fats loves cake, and I suspect he likes it even better when it comes in a package. At Missouri, Fats often brightened up the late afternoon with something called a Boston sundae, which is, more or less, a milkshake with a floating sundae on top—a floating chocolate sundae with bananas if Fats happened to be the customer. I don't mean to imply that Fats was completely undiscriminating. There are good chili dogs and bad chili dogs. The only food that Fats still finds almost literally irresistible is, of course, a double cheeseburger with everything but onions at Winstead's, a hamburger place in Kansas City, and our afflictions differ only in that I prefer the double hamburger with everything and grilled onions. For a number of years, Fats was in the habit of reading the latest diet book at Winstead's—holding the book in one hand and a double cheeseburger with everything but onions in the other.

I didn't see Fats for ten years after college, and when I did see him I didn't recognize him. It was a Sunday morning in New York, and I was at Ratner's on Second Avenue. I was having eggs scrambled with lox and onions, trying to ignore the scoop of mashed potatoes that Ratner's, for some reason, always includes on the plate—perhaps as a way of reminding the customer what less fortunate people may be eating in London, or wherever it's late enough for gentiles to be having dinner. I was glancing around constantly, as I tend to do at Ratner's, to see if some other table was being given a roll basket with more of my favorite kind of onion rolls than our roll basket had. Fats didn't even look familiar. In fact, if we hadn't had some intimate discussions since then about Winstead's hamburgers and Arthur Bryant's barbecued spareribs, I might even now suspect him of being an imposter. Fats later told me that on the morning of May 1, 1959, while employed as a three-hundred-and-twenty-pound salesman of newspaper advertising space in Chicago, he had decided to lose weight. Naturally, he had made similar decisions several dozen times in the past, and he still doesn't know why he was finally able to stop eating. He can't remember any single incident's having set him on his course—no humiliation by some secretary who called him fat stuff, no particularly embarrassing experience buying trousers or trying to tie his shoelace. He is certain that it was not fear for his health that stiffened his will power; several years before, his reaction to a serious warning by a doctor in Kansas City was to think about it over three Winstead's cheeseburgers, a fresh-lime Coke, and a Frosty Malt. On May 1, 1959, Fats started losing weight. He didn't use pills or gimmick diets. "It was cold turkey," he says now, referring to the method rather than the food. "I suffered." In a year, Fats weighed one ninety. Then, gradually, he went down to one sixty. In other words, by the time I saw him at Ratner's the Fats Goldberg I had known was half gone.

Fats was still selling advertising space then, but he wasn't happy in his work. For a while, he tried stand-up comedy, working with a girl in a partnership called Berkowitz and Goldberg—an act that apparently inspired audiences all over town to puzzled silence. Berkowitz and Goldberg finally folded, but fortunately, Fats had one joke left; he opened a restaurant called Goldberg's Pizzeria. He was armed not only with the gimmick of having a Jewish pizza parlor but with the recipe for an excellent version of what the connoisseurs call a Chicago pizza—characterized by a thick, crispy, and particularly fattening crust. I have only an occasional craving for pizza—a craving that I used to nurture carefully, like a small trust fund, at the Spot in New Haven, Connecticut—but I have eaten enough of it to know that Fats serves superior Chicago pizza. Almost as soon as Goldberg's Pizzeria had opened, Fats had what every comic dreams of—a lot of free publicity, critical acclaim, and "exposure" on the *Tonight Show*. (Actually, it was the pizza that was exposed rather than Goldberg; one was given away to a member of the audience who named a tune the band couldn't play.) Fats himself became so celebrated that he was able to publish a pizza cookbook—a volume that may add little to the literature of food but seems at least to have provided a resting place for some old jokes from the Berkowitz and Goldberg days. (One chapter is called "The Goldberg Variations, or How to Make Johann Sebastian Roll Over on His Bach.") Within a few years, there were three Goldberg's Pizzerias, and Fats was getting feelers from conglomerates.

Although Fats enjoys the trappings of a pizza barony, he realizes that his most notable accomplishment is not having created a successful business but having stayed thin. Among his pizza customers are some experts in obesity, and they have informed him that any fat man who remains slim for eighteen years can safely consider himself a medical phenomenon. (Since all Goldberg's Pizzerias display poster-size pictures of Fats when he weighed three cases, the subject of fatness often comes up, particularly on Sunday night, a traditional time for eating pizza and making diet resolutions.) Fats has been told that specialists can always make fat people thin through a variety of hospital treatments—treatments that a layman would probably summarize as solitary confinement. But once released the patients almost invariably become fat again—meaning that, according to any reasonable assessment of the odds, Fats really is someone constantly in danger of weighing three hundred and twenty pounds.

Someone who has gone without a relapse since 1959 is so rare that one researcher from the Rockefeller University asked Fats if he would mind donating some of his fat cells for analysis. Researchers at Rockefeller and at Mt. Sinai Hospital have found that fat people who were fat as children have not only larger fat cells but more of them. When a chronically fat person loses weight, all his fat cells just shrink temporarily, remaining available for re-expansion—or, as someone who apparently enjoys taunting the fatties once put it, "screaming to be refilled." Fat-cell research has led to the depressing speculation that a person who was fat as a child faces horrifying pressure to become fat again and again, no matter how many times he sits in Goldberg's Pizzeria on a Sunday evening and vows that the diet he is going on the following morning will be different. Fats is unenthusiastic about the Rockefeller people's method of studying his fat cells, which would amount to withdrawing a section of tissue from the part of the body in which it is most accessible (or, as Fats sees it, "having three nurses stick an eight-inch needle in my *tushe*") but he sometimes hints that he might be willing to cooperate. The more he thinks about the effort required for a fat man to stay thin, the more he thinks that he is extraordinary enough to be a boon to medical research.

I had a discussion about eating habits with Fats one day at the Gaiety Delicatessen on Lexington Avenue, where he goes every day for a kind of lunchtime breakfast. I ordered the tunafish-salad plate with double coleslaw, hold the potato salad, and a low-caloric cream soda. Fats ate two scrambled eggs, sausages, a bagel with cream cheese, and four cups of coffee with a total of eight packets of sugar. "A fat man's got to have something to look forward to," Fats said. "When I'm reading in bed late at night, I think about being able to have this bagel and cream cheese the next day." Underlying the Fats Goldberg system of weight control is more or less the same philosophy that led to the great Russian purge trials of the thirties—deviation is treason. His Gaiety meals varies daily only in how the eggs are done. In the evening, he has either a steak or half a chicken, baked in the pizza oven. (He is always careful to cut the chicken in half before baking and to put the unneeded half back in the refrigerator. "You have to preplan," he says. "A fat man always cleans his plate.") On Sunday night he permits himself a quarter of a small sausage pizza in place of the steak or chicken, but then he works at the ovens trying to sweat it off. On Monday he cheats to the extent of some bread or maybe a piece of pie. The schedule is maintained only in New York, of course. Kansas City remains a free zone for Fats. He says that in the earlier years of his thinness a week's trip to Kansas City to visit his family would mean gaining seventeen pounds. Lately, restraint has begun to creep into his Kansas City binges. He sometimes manages to visit Kansas City without gaining more than ten pounds.

A few days after our meeting at the Gaiety, Fats happened to drop by my house. It had been a difficult few days for me. St. Anthony's, my favorite Italian street fair, was being held so close to my house that I had been able to convince myself that I could smell the patently irresistible aroma of frying sausages day and night. I have looked all over the country for a sausage I don't like, trying them all along the way. In the course of my research, I have tested country patties in Mississippi and Cuban *chorizos* in Tampa and bratwurst in Yorkville and Swedish potato sausages in Kansas (yes, Kansas) and garlic sausages in Rumanian restaurants in New York and just about everything else that has ever been through a sausage grinder. So far, I love them all. I even like English bangers. I look on the bright side: With all that bread in them, they couldn't possibly cause heartburn. The number of sausage sandwiches I eat at St. Anthony's—Italian sausages that were fried on a griddle right next to the sliced pepper and onion that always accompanies them—is ordinarily limited only by how many *calzones* and *zeppoles* I eat between sausage booths.

Trying, I think, to keep my mind off my own problems, I mentioned to Fats that a doctor I knew had said that in order to gain even fourteen pounds a week in Kansas City it would be necessary for Fats to consume an additional seventy-two hundred calories a day—or the equivalent of fifteen or twenty Winstead's cheeseburgers.

Fats considered that for a while. He didn't seem shocked.

"Just what *did* you eat on a big day in Kansas City the week you gained seventeen pounds?" I asked. I prepared to make a list.

"Well, for breakfast I'd have two eggs, six biscuits with butter and jelly, half a quart of milk, six link sausages, six strips of bacon, and a couple of homemade cinnamon rolls," Fats said. "Then I'd hit MacLean's Bakery. They have a kind of fried cinnamon roll I love. Maybe I'd have two or three of them. Then, on the way downtown to have lunch with somebody, I might stop at Kresge's and have two chili dogs and a couple of root beers. Ever had their chili dogs?"

I shook my head.

"Greasiest chili dogs in the world," Fats said. "I love 'em. Then I'd go to lunch. What I really like for lunch is something like a hot beef sandwich or a hot turkey sandwich. Openfaced, loaded with that flour gravy. With mashed potatoes. Then Dutch apple pie. Kansas City is big on Dutch apple pie. Here they call it apple crumb or something. Then, sometimes in the afternoon, I'd pick up a pie—just an ordinary nine-inch pie—and go to my friend Matt Flynn's house, and we'd cut the pie down the middle and put half in a bowl for each of us and then take a quart of ice cream and cut that down the middle and put it on top of the pie. We'd wash it down with Pepsi-Cola. Sometimes Matt couldn't finish his and I'd have to finish it for him. Then that would be it until I stopped at my sister's house. She's very big on crunchy peanut butter. She even has peanut butter and jelly already mixed. They didn't have that when I was a kid. Then for dinner we'd maybe go to Charlie Bryant's or one of the barbecues out on the highway. At the movies I'd always have a bag of corn and a big Coke and knock off a Payday candy bar. Payday is still my favorite candy bar. They're hard to get here, but they have a very big distribution in Kansas City. Then we'd always end up at Winstead's, of course. Two double cheeseburgers with everything but onions, a fresh-lime Coke and a Frosty Malt. If it was before eleven, I'd stop at the Zarda Dairy for one of their forty-nine-cent banana splits. Then when I'd get home maybe some cherry pie and a sixteen-ounce Pepsi."

And so to bed. I looked at the list. "To tell you the truth, Fats, I'm afraid to add it all up," I said. I looked at the list again. Something on it had reminded me of sausages. It must have been the mention of Bryant's, which used to have barbecue sausages but quit serving them before I had a chance to try them—a situation that has always made me feel like an archeologist who arrived at the tomb just a few days after the locals began to use the best pot for a football. I decided that I would walk over to the fair later and have just one sausage sandwich with peppers and onions—saving a few calories by having a barbecued rather than a fried sausage. If things got out of hand, I figured, I could always go on one of those diets that allow you as much as you want to eat as long as you eat only Brussels sprouts, quinces, and summer squash. I had mentioned the fair to Fats, but he couldn't go. It wasn't a Monday.

"Is life worth living, Fats?" I asked.

"Well, I figure that in my first twenty-five years I ate enough for four normal lifetimes," Fats said. "So I get along. But there is a lot of pain involved. A lot of pain. I can't stress that enough."

CALVIN TRILLIN

ACKNOWLEDGMENTS

Carol Tannenhauser: Who kept repeating that the book was a good idea, a good idea, and without whose foot punching my rear, there would be no book.

Beth Rashbaum, Amanda Vaill, Lindy Hess, Regina Ryan, and **Ilka Shore Cooper:** Five bright and voluptuous editors who took my little hand and led me down the paths of publishing when all I wanted to do was watch the Yankees and "The Rockford Files."

Kate Somers: Voted Most Valuable Researcher by the Fatties of America; who sat in my one-room apartment and wrote the letters, drank Diet Pepsi, made the phone calls, and watched spicy soap operas.

Linda Clement: The biggest Jewish Mother this side of Golda Meir, who talked everyone into sending me stuff.

Osvaldo Mordasini and **Jose Victor Alvarez:** Two mozzarella stars who made the pizzas so I could go home and smack the typewriter around.

Susan Ball: Ace researcher who knew where to dig to get all the hidden poop.

Judy Parelman: One of the greatest phone callers on the banks of the Missouri River.

Pamela Smith: Photo researcher with an eagle eye and the drive of a Mack Truck.

Henry F. Marx and **Cecelia Lazarescu:** The two Kodak Kids who took the before-and-after pictures and didn't even use a wide-angle lens.

Matt Flynn: Very tall hillbilly who is the greatest collector of old advertising and junk in Kansas City.

INTRODUCTION

FATS GOLDBERG'S DIET RIOT

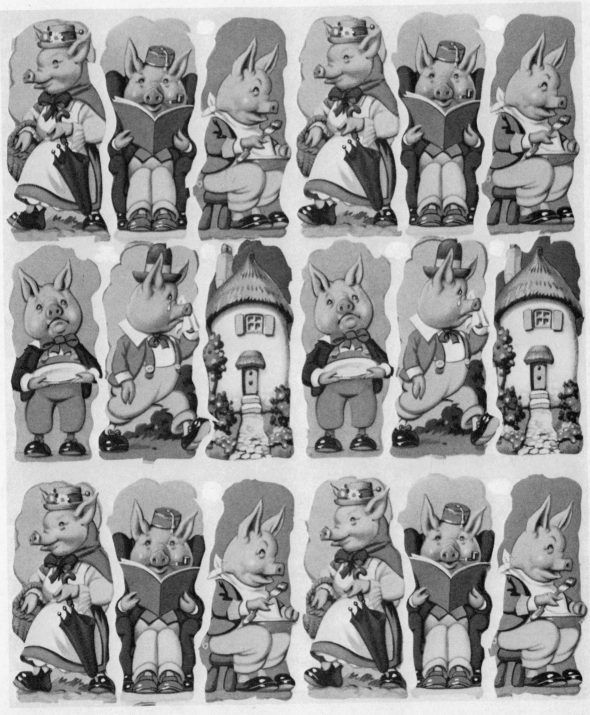

Breakfast: Two scrambled eggs, very soft; three buttermilk pancakes the size of hubcaps; four strips of crisp bacon; four golden-brown link sausages; six homemade biscuits with a quarter pound of butter and half a jar of Smucker's strawberry perserves; half a quart of whole homogenized milk (not that funny, anemic bluish-white stuff they call skim milk); two homemade cinnamon rolls.

Midmorning snack: Two of Kresge's chili dogs; giant foamy root beer.

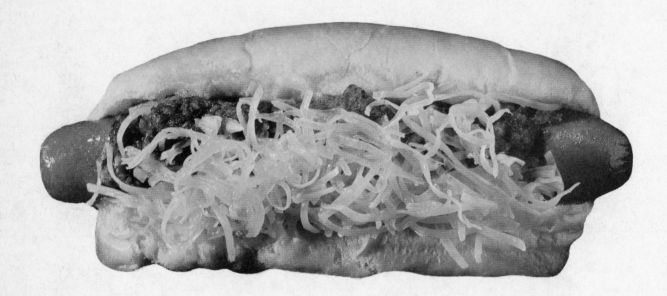

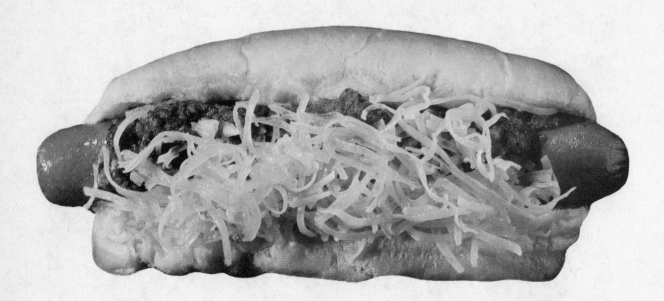

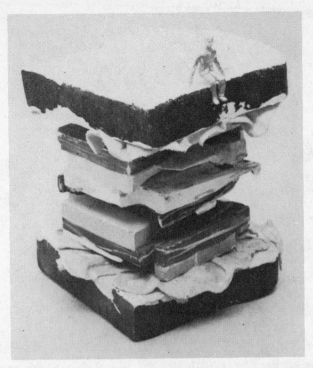

Lunch: Hot roast beef sandwich swimming in thick lumpy beige gravy; three slices of Butternut bread to lap up the gravy; a quarter of a Dutch apple pie, à la mode; two Cokes.

Midafternoon snack: One-half of a fresh banana cake with half a pint of chocolate ice cream.

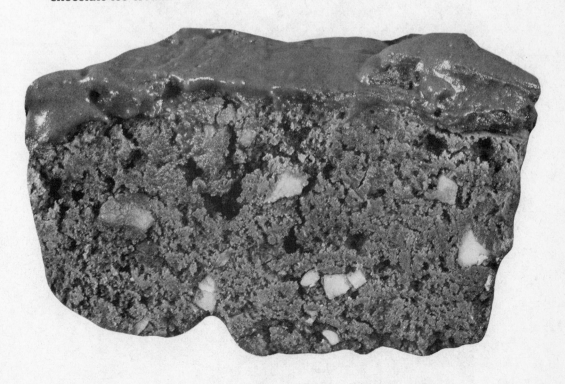

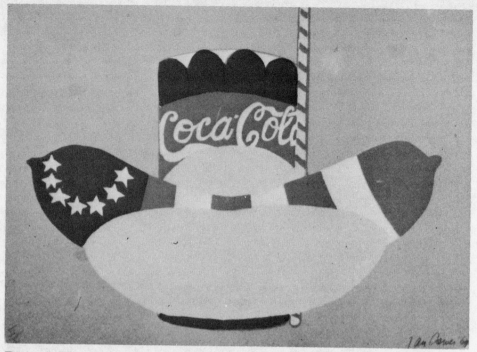

Dinner: Three Winstead's Drive-In double cheeseburgers with everything; order of fries; chocolate Frosty Malt; fresh-lime Coke.

Movie snack: Box of hot buttered popcorn (extra butter, please); large Dr. Pepper; two Payday candy bars.

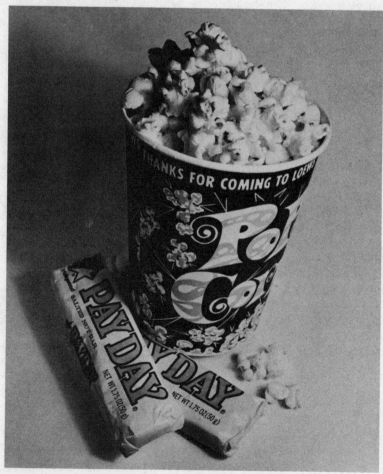

After-movie snack: A 69-cent Zarda Dairy banana split, no maraschino cherries.

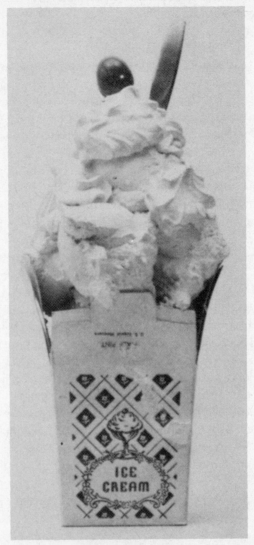

Late-night nosh: Big slice of homemade cherry pie; 16 ounces Pepsi.

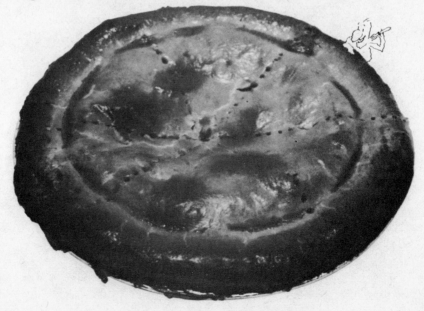

No, this is not what King Kong and Fay Wray ate on the way to the Empire State Building. This is what I ate in one typical day on a recent visit to my home town, Kansas City, Missouri.

In eight gorging days and nine gluttonous nights, I put on a fast eighteen pounds.

Eighteen pound in eight days is a little heartburning even for me, but when I came back to New York, I lost twelve of the eighteen pounds in three weeks.

I do this twice a year. It's good for my soul, but oh, my poor body.

You see, that's me in the photo—the fat, grinning Buddha with the large earlobes. Or rather, that *was* me, 18 years ago when I weighed an incredible 320 pounds. The slim matinée idol is me too—last month when I slipped in at 160 pounds. I had lost a whole Goldberg. But the monster's ready to come back to life any time I slide back to my old gorging habits.

I am a foodaholic. I mainline Mallomars. I'm a Chunky junkie. Even the word "food" conjures up mouth-watering dreams of hot drippy pepperoni pizza, huge Cokes with crushed ice, crisp crinkly French fries, so greasy my fingers are slick, and thick chocolate shakes with little lumps of vanilla ice cream still floating around.

Nothing used to get between me and food. When I was twenty-two and had just graduated from college, I had a complete physical, the first one of my life. After putting me through some horrible tests, the doctor took me into his office, shut the door, and announced that I had diabetes (of the latent variety—but quite real enough for me). My three double chins started to tremble; I was terrified. But, he said, I could control my diabetes through diet. I regained my composure, walked out the door, got in my car and drove to NuWay Drive In, and ate three hotdogs, potato salad, and a chocolate shake. When I was fat and got hungry, the angel of death could be sitting on my shoulder and I wouldn't miss a bite.

Very funny. Unfortunately for most fatties, it's the old story of laughing through the tears. And the world doesn't make it any easier. First of all, I have to eat every day to live. Even worse, when I walk down any street, I see and smell delicatessens, pizza stands, Baskin-Robbinses, and the hot pretzel pusher. Food is all around us.

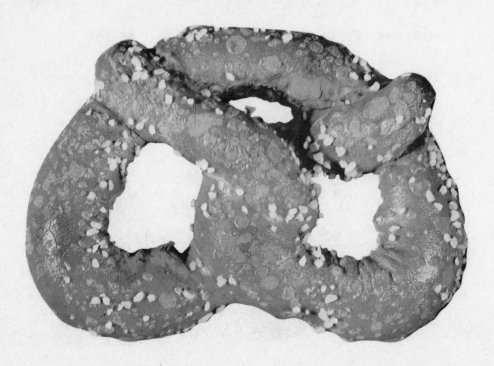

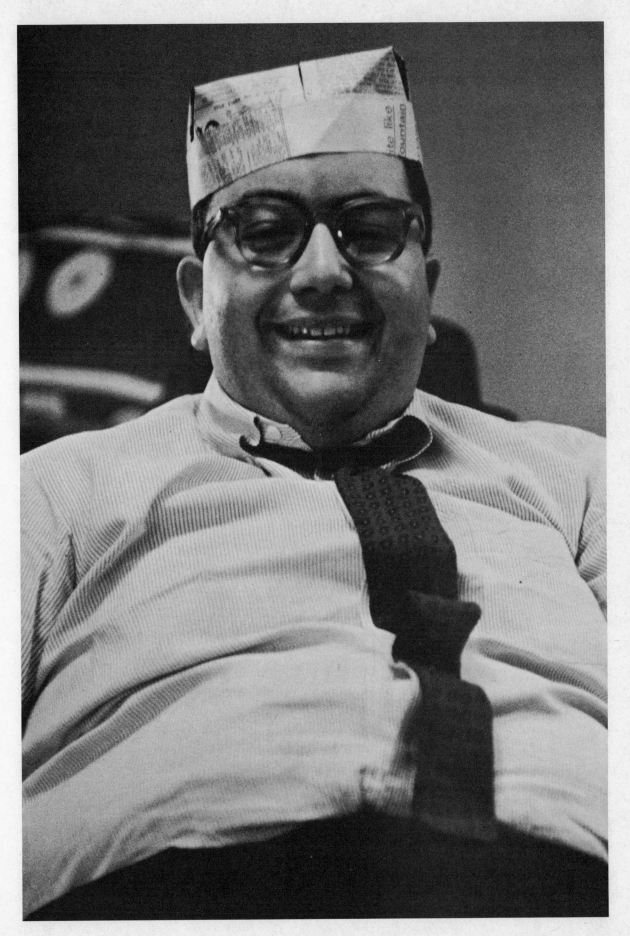

And there is no way a food addict can get a nonfattening fix. I walked through my local supermarket and proved that, for a buck, I could gobble either five pounds of bananas, or two big bags of potato chips, or one and a half pecan coffee cakes, or six Eskimo Pies, or nine Twinkies, or 54 Oreo Creme Sandwiches, or a jar of Skippy peanut butter, a jar of grape jelly, and a loaf of Wonder bread. But there are virtually no nonfattening snacks that I can buy and eat on the run. If I can't get—or don't want—foods like fruit or pickles, I have to chew my knuckles.

How did I get into this bind? When I was born, forty-three years ago, to Sara and Art Goldberg of Kansas City, Missouri, I weighed 7 pounds 14 ounces. Sara, who weighs 140 pounds, is the Jelly Bean Queen of K.C. She still hangs around Woolworth's candy counter eating candy orange slices. Art weighed 150 pounds, never got hungry, and owned a food emporium called, not surprisingly, Goldberg's Market—"Fancy Groceries and Meats," with free delivery. (I was the free delivery.) Jocelyn, my sister, is five years older than me . . . and skinny. Lucky Joc.

Ma says I was a "chunky" baby and that I was eating everything in sight while I was still gurgling in her arms. By sixth grade, I weighed a cool 200 pounds. When Ma would cook she'd make six pork chops; one for each of them and three for me. I was so "chunky" I couldn't sit in a normal desk. Mrs. Burns, my teacher, had me sit in a straight chair on the side of the room.

My pediatrician once hauled me up on the table when I was a little fat kid and said, "Do you want to die in ten years?" I tipped in at 240 in the eighth grade. After I waddled to three doctors, they diagnosed my malady as a severe case of overeating. This is when the diets started. Every doctor would gaze at my stomach and give me a mimeographed sheet with sample diets for seven days. You know the kind: breakfast was half an orange, a poached egg, a slice of dry toast, and half a glass of skim milk. Lunch and dinner were just as boring. I'd bring the diet home, diet through breakfast, and blow the whole deal at lunch.

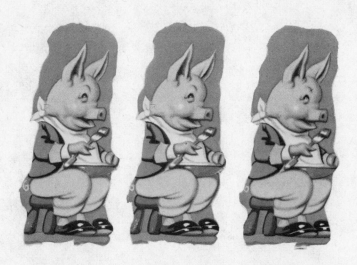

My parents couldn't stop me from eating—no parents could. They'd have had to keep an eye on me twenty-four hours a day. If I couldn't eat at home or in the gorcery store stockroom, I'd eat at neighbors', friends', strangers', or any place where I found a spare cashew.

Popping diet pills came during my freshman year at high school. It started with one pill a half hour before each meal, each pill a different color. I ran the whole diet pill string, from the worthless ones through the powerful Dexedrine spansules that made me giggle a lot. None worked for long. The minute I'd stop taking the pills, I'd start eating all over again. The only real difference in my life was that now I was terrified all the time, a perpetual hypochondriac.

High school was a lot of laughs. I bought a '37 Oldsmobile that started leaning toward the left. Anyone who sat next to me automatically slid down to my side on the nylon seat cover. That could have been exciting, except I had only two dates in high school. Both were with the same girl on consecutive New Year's Eves. Four friends and I were supposed to go out stag. But both times they got dates and fixed me up without telling me, until they surprised me on the big night. They knew I wouldn't have gone if I'd known. I was plenty mad and also plenty scared.

Actually, there was one other date in high school—the Sunday school confirmation dance. Everyone in the class had dates except me and Lucille Soberman. Poor Lucy was almost as fat as I was, so the Sunday school teacher arranged the fix-up. That was one of the worst evenings, I'm sure, that either of us had spent in our entire lives. We just hung around the refreshment table the entire evening. The amounts we ate were about even, but I think she may have outdone me a little. We danced once. That was the first time I'd ever held a girl in my arms— also the first time I'd ever danced. But we were so big our extended arms could barely touch each other's sides. You should have seen us cha-cha.

My official weight when I graduated from high school and got my draft card was 265 pounds. Kansas City Junior College was next.

During my first year there I sold ladies' shoes at a local Baker's Shoe Store and got my nickname of "Three Cases Goldberg." Selling a "case" in shoe peddling means selling $100 worth of shoes. For me, though, the name applied not to my sales, but to my size—300-pound Goldberg.

In college guys are supposed to become clothes-conscious, but I did all my Beau Brummell work at either Sears or the local army-navy store. These were the only places that could fit me. My costume never varied. First I wore Sears Roebuck's "Armored Crotch" boxer shorts—I could swear that was the brand name. They were reinforced between the legs because you know how fat boys chafe. Then I wore size 17½ white or blue oxford-cloth button-down shirts, and overall pants with a hammer pocket that hung rakishly under my tummy. I was a 300-pound sex bomb with saddle shoes.

When I moved on to the University of Missouri to study journalism, I pledged Zeta Beta Tau fraternity. There I went formal and switched to 48-inch-waist khakis instead of the overalls. I now weighed 305 pounds, and had managed to kiss one girl, once.

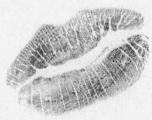

I always tried to take a shower alone in the fraternity house because I was embarrassed by my size. One day I happened to glance at my naked body after taking a shower. I noticed a string of little red scratches circling my tummy. Although I tried never to look at myself completely undressed, now that I had done so, panic set in. I ran to the doctor, who told me those red lines were stretch marks. That is, the skin couldn't hold the fat. He reassured me that they were harmless and that pregnant women get them all the time. But, I whimpered, I wasn't a pregnant woman. I was thoroughly depressed until I could get to a pint of butterscotch swirl ice cream.

Once during my first year, after I had eaten three complete lunches in one hour, I thought I had finally done it: I was going to die from overeating. Struggling over to the infirmary, I bared my soul to the doctor. I begged him for a diet. Being more accustomed to mononucleosis than to cases such as mine, he pushed his finger in my stomach, shook his head, told me to cool it on the groceries, gave me a can of foot powder, and sent me home. He didn't realize he was dealing with an addict—and what an addict!

The worst night I ever spent during my fat years was in the fraternity house, two months before graduation. As usual, after my customary three-and-a-half portion dinner, I started to watch TV or thumb through a book. And—again as usual—I started salivating around eight thirty, waiting for the sandwich man who came around at ten o'clock. But that night he didn't show. By eleven thirty I was in a state of panic. Everything was closed except for the highway cafés and the doughnut shop in downtown Columbia, and to top it all off, it was snowing. I ran from room to room, sweating and screaming for someone to take me to eat. At last, Dave Goodman, God bless him, took pity on my crazed condition and drove me to the Broadway Donut Shop; after a dozen hot glazed doughnuts and a quart of chocolate milk, I finally stopped twitching.

After I graduated from college in journalism, I had four jobs that first year. I counted Japanese thong sandals in bins, sold radio time for a rock station in K.C., went back to Columbia, Missouri, as a radio announcer (calling myself Fats Goldberg, the Sheik of Columbia), and was a television announcer, off camera, of course. Finally I wound up in Chicago working for the *Chicago Tribune,* and it was there that I made a decision. I was tired of being fat. It was ugly and uncomfortable, the morning heartburn really hurt, and being fat was rapidly becoming a lot less funny than it had once seemed.

So on Monday, May 1, 1959, I awoke and rubbed my food-swollen eyes and said to myself, "Today's the day I'm going to start my diet." I'd said those words to myself almost every morning since the day I was born. But this was *it.*

The last time I'd weighed myself was three or four months before when I'd found a freight and cattle scale. (Household scales, at least the ones I've seen, go only to 300 pounds.) I hopped on the freight scale, and when the needle started careening over 300 and wasn't slowing down, I leaped off. It had hit 320.

On the first day of the rest of my life, I literally rolled out of bed and took a Dexedrine spansule diet pill. After a breakfast of two scrambled eggs, an English muffin, and two cups of coffee, I decided there'd be no more diet pills for me. Either I was going to do this cold turkey, just me and my stomach, or I'd just keep eating until my navel popped out and I'd die, having lived a short fat life.

For lunch, I had to meet a car dealer to whom I was trying to sell ad space in the *Tribune,* and he wanted to go to a smorgasbord. What a way to start a diet! But I ate only a couple of pieces of roast beef and a few green beans. And for dinner I held myself to steak and cottage cheese.

The first three letters of *diet,* as was pointed out in something I once read, are *die.* By my second day of dieting, I believed death would have been easier. I didn't think I could take dieting any longer. With no exaggeration, my whole body from my hair to my corns craved and demanded food. Still, I gritted my underused teeth and somehow stuck it out.

At 320 pounds, 190 was my goal, but it seemed to be a lifetime away. It took me twenty-five years to put that weight on and I wanted to take it off in three days. The second week I lost seventeen pounds. I didn't care if it was water or cheesecake, I was losing weight. This made me feel great. I was accomplishing something. I could feel it and I could see it when I got on the scale.

When I made that decision to diet, I had to make a total commitment to a new life-style. If I was going to lose weight, I had to stop eating. So when the hunger pains were making my stomach do the Charleston, I would think about Caterpillar tractors, joint sessions of Congress, Marilyn Monroe—anything except food.

Somewhere along the line, I read that the proper way to eat was to breakfast like a king, lunch like a prince, and dine like a pauper. I've used that system for years and it works, though I've now developed Goldberg's variations on it, about which you will hear more later. At that time, I would get up in the morning, drink a glass of skim milk to get me rolling, then follow it with two eggs, toast, and coffee. Sometimes I'd throw in a little bacon or sausage. Lunch was a sandwich and a glass of skim milk. I always took the top piece of bread off and folded the two halves together. That way I saved the calories in a slice of bread. Dinner was meat of some kind, or chicken or turkey, with cottage cheese or tomato.

One of the hardest things for me to learn was how to add variety to my diet. I used to find a food that would let me lose weight and I'd eat so much of it, I'd get to the point where I couldn't stand to look at it any more. Fresh pineapple is one example. It was juicy, cold, and sweet, and it filled me up. But I ate so much, leaves almost started growing out of my head. Boredom is a dangerous feeling when you're dieting.

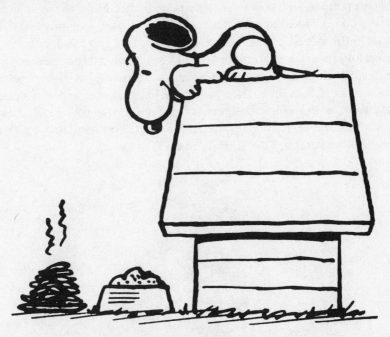

Happiness is a side dish of French-fries.

Copr. © 1958 United Feature Syndicate, Inc.

My over-all goal was to lose 130 of my 320 pounds, but being weak and not knowing how long I could last without a food reward, I set intermediate goals. The first goal was to weigh 265 pounds when I went on vacation to Kansas City, after three months of dieting. When I walked in the back door of my house, Ma was peeling potatoes. She looked up and said, "Yes?" For a second, she hadn't even recognized her bouncing baby boy. I was thrilled.

Everywhere, in Chicago and K.C., people would notice the difference immediately. My size 52-long suits were getting very baggy. I woke up without heartburn. Everyone was tremendously encouraging and when they got me alone, would ask how I did it. The management at the *Chicago Tribune* became more interested in my career. I was taken off probation on the company's major medical policy. I developed a new self-confidence and outlook on everything, including my social life.

Demon temptations were always around: pungent-smelling fast-food joints, or dinner in a restaurant or someone's house. But I learned how to cope by saying *No*.

Pain was still my constant companion—the physical pain of being hungry and the psychological pain of deprivation. I had to change my life-style to one that wasn't centered around food.

And I did it. In one year I lost 130 pounds.

It was at that point, when I weighed 190 pounds, that I went into the pizza business. I figured that if I couldn't eat it, I could become a pizza voyeur and sell and smell it. Suddenly, at the age of thirty-four, I was standing in front of two 650-degree ovens schlepping pizzas. It was like working in front of a Gary, Indiana, open hearth. The old scale started going down again. Terrific. Now, nine years later, I'm 160 pounds and lean like a cougar.

In the last few years, I've developed the Goldberg Oasis Method of Maintenance. I eat everything I want on Monday night, storing up food like a camel. Then I diet Tuesday and Wednesday. Thursday I have another eating orgy, to carry me through the diet days of Friday, Saturday, and Sunday. On a Monday or Thursday it's nothing for me to put on five pounds. But I take those pounds right off on my diet days. I have to have those two binge days to look forward to—each is an oasis in the middle of the diet desert.

Except for Monday and Thursday, my life is cemented into a routine. I eat two meals a day. Since my work at the pizza stands is primarily at night, I get up late and have a glass of skim milk. Then I work the lunch shift at one of the pizzerias. About 2:00 P.M., at the Gaiety Delicatessen, I have a large brunch of soft scrambled eggs with sausage, bacon, or pastrami, a toasted buttered bagel with a little cream cheese, and coffee. This is my food thrill of the day.

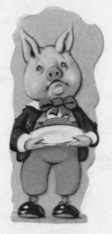

For dinner I have yogurt with bran, half a chicken, or four ounces of roast beef, plus a little salad and fruit. By 11 o'clock I'm against the wall with hunger. Sometimes it gets so bad that I can't wait to brush my teeth, so I can at least get the taste of Crest toothpaste.

I also dream of food. (I have this recurring dream of bakeries. . . .) Sometimes I wake up feeling sorry for myself. But I have twenty-five years of outstanding eating behind me, and I remind myself that I probably ate more in those twenty-five years than a normal person would eat in a lifetime. I feel better when I look at it that way.

For years, I saw myself as a trim Burt Lancaster or a rugged Gary Cooper. Right now I'm svelte, but I'll never be rugged. And as for shoulders, I didn't come equipped with any. My formal exercise is limited to a little yoga—shoulder stands (possible even on my meager shoulders) to save my hair. I also do lots of walking—a fast two or three miles a day on the hot New York concrete. This keeps me in pretty good shape, and keeps my podiatrist happy.

During my first year of dieting, I developed "Dr." Goldberg's Diet Dicta:

1. Find what works for *you*. The reducing Golden Rule is: Anything that works, is good. When you find it, fit it into your life-style.
2. Be flexible. Add variety.
3. Don't eat fattening foods.
4. Eat a balanced diet.
5. Eat slowly. Put the fork *down* after every bite. Before I lost weight, I ate like a windmill—just one whirling, continuous circular motion from the plate to my mouth and back again.
6. See your doctor before going on any diet.

I contemplated, mused, and daydreamed for twenty-five years, but in the end I learned there's only one way to lose weight. I had to change the way I lived. I determined to try not to eat fattening foods and to eat a balanced diet. And I succeeded.

There you have it—the way I live and diet. The diet path I've chosen works for me. My fat outlook on life has changed to thin. I am finally a "normal" person, though "normality" was a shock at first.

As a fat man I was safe. That big wall of fat protected me. While other kids were going through the trials of puberty and dating, I escaped by eating my way through adolescence. No wonder I didn't go through puberty until I was thirty-one. No one could get close to me, literally or figuratively. Kidding and teasing were important to keep people away. But now that I'm thin, I don't have to hide behind my fat. I'm more honest about how I feel. And this gives me something I never had—self-confidence. I have become more relaxed and self-assured. Other people look at me with respect, which is a totally new sensation.

After going through the disciplines of dieting, I feel there is nothing I can't handle.

In my B.C. (Before Counting) days, I couldn't call a woman for a date without the phone sliding out of my sweaty hand. Not that I became a swaggering boulevardier or a Robert Redford overnight, but now I can get up the courage to approach a woman.

There are also other big bonuses. I can go into Brooks Brothers without the salesman giggling, snorting, and hiding behind the crew-neck sweaters. I can sleep on my stomach without having a stomachache in the morning. I've stopped gnawing my fingernails. I can wear La Costa knit shirts without looking like two St. Bernards in a bag fighting to get out. I have a hundred times more energy and require three hours less sleep. Ties don't have to be extra long to fit around my 17½-inch neck. I can tie my shoes without crossing my legs. I can sit in a movie theater seat straight and not on my side. People will sit next to me on the bus. I don't perspire as much. Women look at me admiringly on the street. Clothes don't wear out as fast. I can see and feel my bones. I can get in and out of the smallest cars. I even bought a Volkswagen. I have stopped snoring. Sometimes someone says I am too thin and should eat more. I can be the last one on a crowded elevator.

AND if I live even one minute longer because I lost weight, it was all worth it.

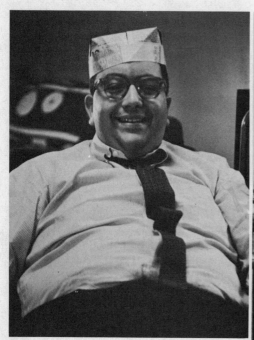

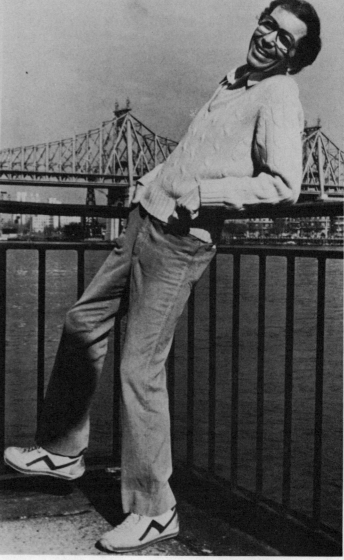

A THIN AUTHOR'S NOTE

As you're reading this massive volume of dieting information, you're probably either getting hungry or wondering how I ever got this book together.

All the poop here was gotten through public information sources. I started with the telephone directories of the thirty largest cities in the United States. I then went to government sources, trade associations and magazines, insurance companies, the travel industry, newspapers, magazines, television, radio, medical sources, friends, enemies, strangers, or any other source or person who could give me a scrap of information on losing weight.

All of the sources were sent two personal letters followed up by a personal phone call. There are no value judgments on any of the information in the Catalog. I'm not a member of the C.I.A., so there was no spying or undercover work. Anyone who did not want to be here was not included, or was simply mentioned among the city-by-city listings at the back of the book.

What you hold in your hands, therefore, is every scrap of diet information I could lay my hands on.

If you have any additional or more up-to-date information, if you have been omitted from the listings and would now like to be included, if you have any suggestions or criticisms, or even if you would only like to write me a torrid love letter, please, please drop me a note at Macmillan Publishing Company, 866 Third Avenue, New York, New York 10022.

HOW TO USE THIS BOOK

We are all individuals, with different tastes, appetites, and life-styles. Therefore any diet that will help *you* lose weight and keep it off must fit into *your* personal life-plan. With this book, you can pick and choose from a lot of diet information and develop your own system, as I did. Or you can go to a diet group meeting, read a book, go to a fat farm, or attend any number of diet courses, and find that a particular diet or system works for you in its entirety. What this book is really like (sorry to mention it in a diet book) is a smorgasbord: you can eat one food (or stick with one diet plan) until your ears fall off, or you can fill your plate with fifty things.

Of course, I'm still looking for that one magic elixir that will automatically make me thin forever without my having to give up one French fry; but with one large salty tear trickling down my rosy cheek, I'm sorry to report that, after all this research, I haven't found it.

The only way to lose weight is to eat less and exercise more—to keep burning up calories faster than you take them in. I hope this book helps you find the right system for you.

MY DOCTOR SPEAKS

I have had Larry Goldberg as a patient for many years. Although he wasn't my patient when he was losing, he has maintained his present weight for the nine years that I have seen him. In fact, he is twenty pounds less than when I first saw him in 1968. Goldberg is somewhat of a medical rarity, in that he has learned that obesity is a constant lifelong battle. A battle that he knows is never won completely.

Obesity is a critical disease that has to be controlled. By now, you know some of the medical dangers of being overweight; coronary problems, diabetes and high blood pressure.

He has convinced me that success in weight reduction is an individual success. You and you alone must be responsible for the way you live and eat. You have to devise your own weight reduction program based on your individual needs, behavior and habits.

Goldberg has compiled this catalog to help you find the best method for yourself. I must warn you to be careful. Some of the methods are medically proven. Some are not. Some are plain common sense. Some are pure speculation and risky. Whatever you try, consult your family doctor first.

I wish you success.

Martin E. Bloomfield, M.D.
New York City

YOU'D BETTER READ THIS

I'm taking one whole page—and pages cost much money—to tell you something. No, more than tell you—beseech you, command you. And you'd better damn well do what I tell you!

Before you do anything in the weight-reducing field or try any of the products or projects mentioned in this book:

GO TO YOUR DOCTOR AND DISCUSS THE DIET WITH HIM!

I'm going to repeat this throughout the book until you're sick of it, but it's *your* health I'm worried about.

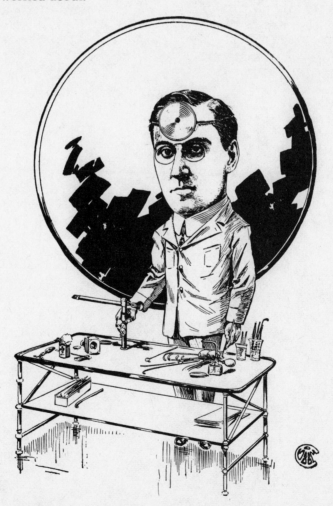

P.S. I do not work for the American Medical Association.

SACCHARIN COULD GET THE SACK

As this magnificent specimen of a book is struggling to the press, the Food and Drug Administration has announced the ban of saccharin from the market.

Since many food and drink products mentioned here do contain saccharin, and since it is not clear at this writing whether or not the ban will be sustained, I recommend that you check the label of any dietetic product you might want to buy.

ONE

DIET BOOKS

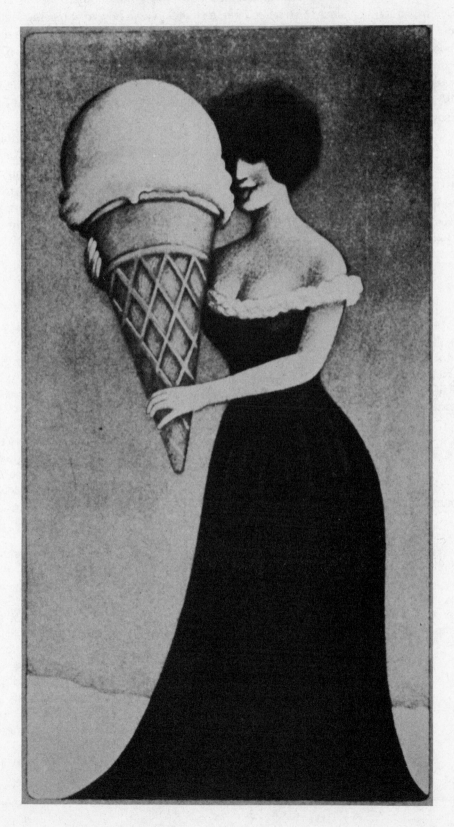

Read 'em and Weep

I'm hooked on diet books. When I go into any bookstore, I head straight for the diet and health section.

I have yet to read a diet book that I don't get a little something out of—whether it's a new place to sit when I eat, a suggestion on how to eat, some medical knowledge, or the calorie count of Snickers candy bars. The best gimmick diet book and the funniest diet book I ever read was one of the first I laid eyes on. It came out about the late 1940s, and was reissued by Paperback Library in 1968. It was called *The Fat Boy Book* and the author was a super salesman named Elmer Wheeler. This book was so popular that restaurants in Kansas City featured Fat Boy Menus.

Of course, like all books, some diet books are outstanding, some are terrible, and many are in between. I've tried to cover the whole range of diet books, from the ridiculous to the classic. But read them with care, because a diet book can do harm, too. Make sure what it tells you is right for you—that's the reason why I emphasize that you should see your doctor. Just because you laid out a couple of bucks for a weight-reducing book, doesn't mean you have to go immediately on the diet. Take it easy, think about it, and keep reading.

All the publishers' addresses are listed at the end of the book.

**CONSUMER GUIDE
RATING THE DIETS
by Theodore Berland and the Editors of
    Consumer Guide
$1.95 Paperback 322 pages
    Publications International Ltd.**

Before you get started on any diet regimen you should check out the competition, and to do this you absolutely must have *Rating the Diets*: 322 pages of the best weight-control information you'll ever find. As its title implies, the book discusses the pros and cons of almost every diet you've ever heard of—from Weight Watchers through the banana and milk diet. The authors also discuss the physiological and psychological aspects of overweight, and there's some fascinating information on what happens to food when you eat it, as well as on what happens when you diet.

**THE TRUTH ABOUT WEIGHT
CONTROL
by Neil Solomon, M.D., with Sally
    Sheppard
$1.50 Paperback 300 pages Dell
    Books**

This is a complete introduction to the art and science of dieting and one of the best diet books around. Done in a question-and-answer format, it has twenty chapters on such subjects as "Instant Beginnings, or, What You Can Do Right Now," "What Is a Fad Diet?" and "Diet Clubs."

Dr. Solomon has long been a practitioner in the field of weight control. He teaches at Johns Hopkins University Medical School, and is Maryland's Secretary of Health and Mental Hygiene. He is also the originator of the term "Yo-Yo Syndrome"—an expression that refers to those people who are forever losing weight and putting it back on, or going up and down. The Yo-Yo Syndrome has been installed in the permanent diet vernacular, and Dr. Solomon devotes a chapter to it here.

The whole book is a treasure trove of dieting information—there's no baloney in it, just good hard facts.

"System" Diets

System diet books sell the best, so of course there are more of them than of any other group of diet books. A good system diet book takes you by your pudgy hand and leads you step by step through the entire process of losing weight. It tells you what to eat, how to eat, and the results you'll get if you follow the "system."

The systems vary according to the person writing the book and are generally devised by doctors. Take a look and pick out the system that could work on your system.

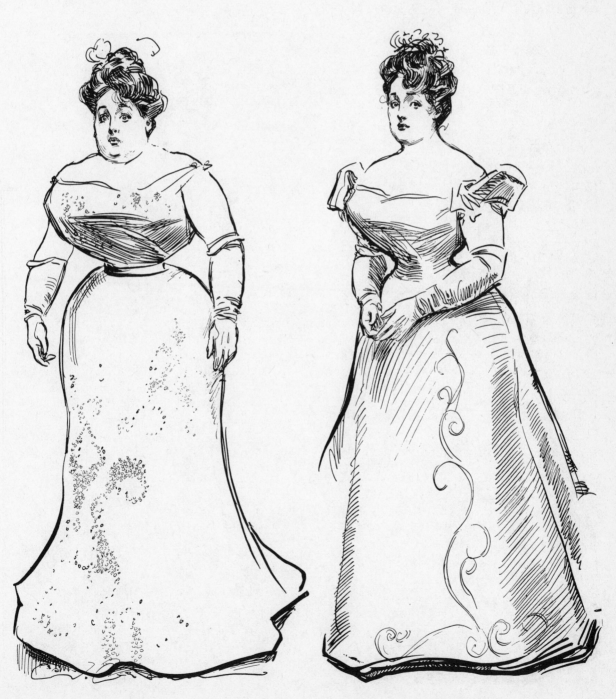

Calorie-Counting

REDUCE WITH THE LOW CALORIE DIET
by Marvin Small
$1.50 Paperback 287 pages Pocket Books

This is among the most basic diet books. *Reduce with the Low Calorie Diet* first came out in 1953 and has gone through twenty-five printings—which should tell you something. Twenty-four years is a long life for a diet book.

The book offers no gimmicks, just a straight, low-calorie diet plus a snap-out calorie-counter to carry in your pocket. Most of the book is taken up with tempting low-calorie recipes for over 400 foods. Illustrated.

If you've never bought a diet book, this could be the one to get you off on your skinny journey.

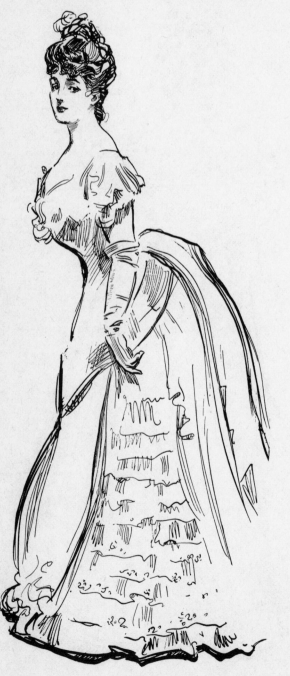
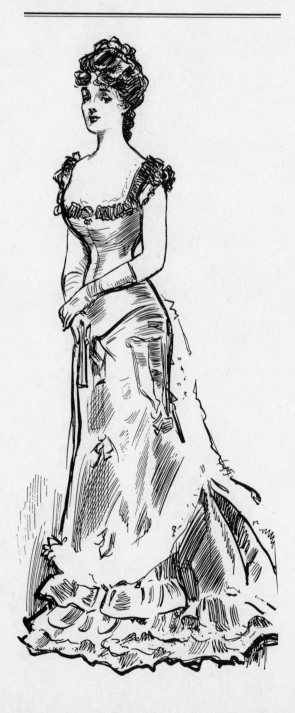

THE PRUDENT DIET
by Iva Bennett and Martha Simon
$1.95 Paperback 335 pages Bantam Books

This is the granddaddy of all diets and diet books: the Prudent Diet has probably been copied, modified, and used by more people and groups than any other diet on the overweight horizon.

On the cover of the book it says, "Based on 14 years of research of the Nutrition Bureau, New York City Department of Health, the Prudent Diet not only decreases blood cholesterol, but also lowers blood pressure and blood sugar levels, decreases body weight and reduces the rate of heart attacks by more than 50%." Those are some heavy claims, but the authors offer data to prove them.

Dr. Norman Jolliffe, Director of the Nutrition Bureau, started using the Prudent Diet in 1957 with his Anti-Coronary Club. This was a group of 1000 men in their fifties who were likely candidates for heart trouble.

The Prudent Diet reduces the quantity of calories, cholesterol and saturated fat in your diet. Instead of counting calories, you weigh your food, choosing foods from among six groups containing the key nutrients.

1. Fish, meat, poultry and eggs—for protein, iron, and B-vitamins.
   Fish and shellfish must be eaten at least five times a week, at any meal. Meats must be limited to sixteen ounces per week, in four-ounce portions. Poultry—any kind you want—should be eaten often. Eggs are limited to four per week for adults.
2. Milk and dairy products—for calcium, riboflavin, and protein.
   Type and amount varies with adults and children. But avoid butter, cream cheese, and ice cream.
3. Dark green, leafy, and deep yellow vegetables—for Vitamin A.
   At least three to four servings per week.
4. Fruits—for Vitamin C.
   A specified selection that you can choose from and eat a lot of daily.
5. Breads and cereals—for B-vitamins, iron, and calories.
   Whole grains must be eaten at every meal. You should avoid cakes, cookies, and pastries. They're loaded with saturated fats.
6. Vegetables, oils, and margarines containing polyunsaturated fats.
   A specified amount each day but avoid butter and lard.

If the Prudent Diet sounds familiar, it should be. Jean Nidetch used the New York Health Department diet when she started Weight Watchers, and all the groups that copied W.W. have used diets similar to this one.

The book also contains many recipes and menu plans.

The philosophy of the Prudent Diet is best expressed by the authors: "Dr. Norman Jolliffe called the diet 'prudent' because the word means sensible or wise. In brief, the Prudent Diet is a well-balanced diet, designed to promote positive health and to prolong the vigorous span of life. The Prudent Diet advocates neither excessive use of nor complete omission of any one food."

Unfortunately, the only place you can get this kind of sound advice is between the covers of this book. Dr. Norman Jolliffe died in 1961, and because of the financial woes of New York City there is no more Anti-Coronary Club nor are there any New York City Obesity Clinics.

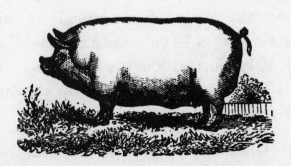

DOCTOR SOLOMON'S EASY, NO-RISK DIET
by Neil Solomon, M.D., Ph.D., and Mary Knudson
$1.95 Paperback 240 pages Warner Books

Dr. Solomon is the author of the best-selling *The Truth About Weight Control* (see p. 2), and in this book he has come up with a specific diet to help you lose weight.

The Easy, No-Risk Diet is a 1200-calorie diet, but you won't be counting calories. Dr. Solomon has done it for you. This is an exchange diet: there are lists of the foods you *may* eat, from which you choose which ones you *will* eat. As Dr. Solomon says, "Any food on the list has the same caloric content as any other food on the list. The choice is yours." Flexibility and variety are the key words, so you won't get bored and start stuffing yourself again.

You must eat a certain number of shares in the following categories: protein foods, dairy foods, fruits, breads, and vegetables. You also may substitute such goodies as pretzels, ice cream, or half a bagel.

There are also suggested daily menus, a section on how to prepare foods, an Easy, No-Risk Diet for "Carboholics," and a "Minidiet—for Working People Who Won't Take Time to Diet."

A special feature of the book is Chapter 6: "Diet Meditation ('DM')—How to Stay on Your Diet." Dr. Solomon tells you to work on your subconscious with a process known as affirmative automatic response, which involves positive suggestion and keeping a daily diary. This is the first diet guru I've encountered. But he takes you through all the steps, so don't be scared.

THE NIBBLER'S DIET
by Pat Hunter
$1.00 Paperback 128 pages Essendess Special Editions

The nibbles in the Nibbler's Diet are foods like lettuce, mustard greens, and bean sprouts—so don't get excited thinking that you're going to be nibbling cashew nuts and bowls of hot buttered popcorn.

Every pound contains 3500 calories. To lose one pound a day means giving up 3500 calories a day. To lose 3500 calories requires three hours of running. If you walk, you're using up five or six calories a minute. If you bicycle, it's eight calories a minute. Swimming is 11 calories a minute, and running is 19 calories a minute. If you eat a large apple, 101 calories, you lose the calories it contains by walking 19 minutes, biking 12 minutes, swimming 9 minutes, or running 5 minutes.

Pat Hunter was given this diet by a doctor in 1954, when he discovered she had a low-blood-sugar problem. She lost about thirty-five pounds on this diet and then forgot about it. She found the diet again several years later, when she was cleaning out her diet drawer.

Basically this is just another low-calorie regimen, but with one small difference: you eat a low-calorie breakfast, lunch, and dinner, but in between you can eat all the specified nibbles you want to ward off those awful hunger pangs. To make it all easy, Ms. Hunter gives you six weeks of dinner menus and an exceptionally good low-calorie recipe section—including recipes for such exotic foods as Butterfly Shrimp and Charlotte Russe—that is a large part of the book.

THE 100 CALORIE MIRACLE DIET
by Bunny Yeager
$1.50 Paperback 186 pages Pinnacle Books

Hey guys, the cover of this book is the diet's best recommendation: a shot of Bunny Yeager stretched out on the grass in a hot-stuff bikini.

(And inside there are sixteen pages showing her doing exercises in a leotard.)

But back to the diet. The gimmick in the "100 Calorie Miracle Diet" is that you're never to eat more than 100 calories at one time. Of course, Ms. Yeager says you must eat sixteen times a day. Therefore you're never consuming over 1600 calories a day, which is what most low-calorie diets call for. Let's take some examples from her "Rich Man's Luxury Diet."

1. half a cheese blintz (76 calories)
   one-third cup fresh diced cantaloupe (24 calories)
   one cup black coffee
2. six macadamia nuts (90 calories)
3. half a fresh mango (90 calories)
   one Social Tea cookie (21 calories)

And so on for sixteen meals a day. There are also about 100 pages of sample menus and calorie-counts of foods 100 calories or less. What it is, is a snack diet. Or as they say in New York, you nosh a lot.

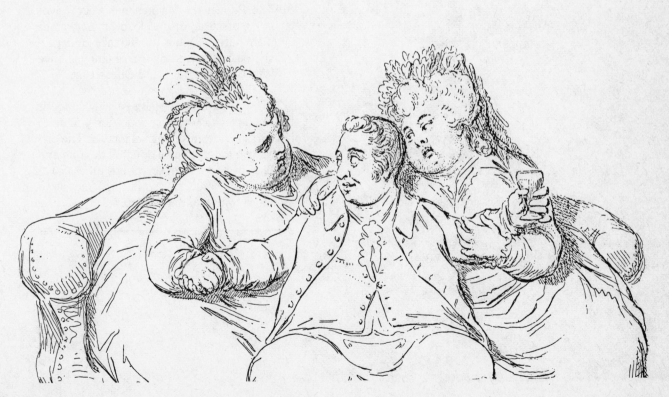

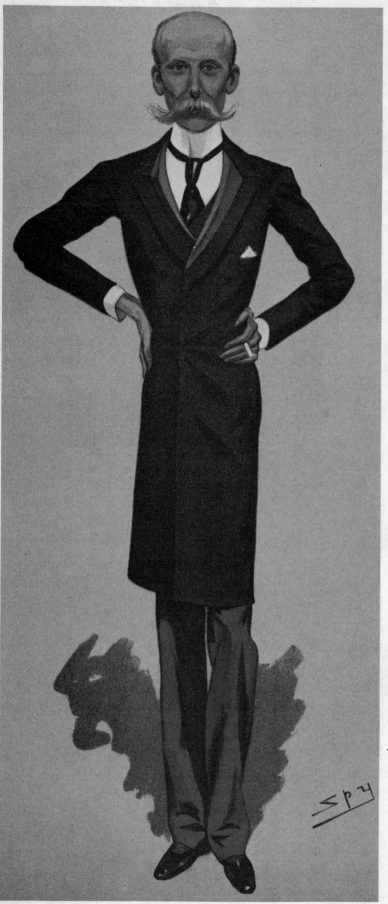

DIET CYBERNETICS FOR LEAN LINES
by Antonio S. Marotta and Lorraine Fay Wurtzel
$1.25 Paperback 173 pages Pyramid Books

Like *Slim Forever* (see p. 11), *Diet Cybernetics* complements the program of a diet group—in this case Lean Lines, which operates throughout New Jersey, New York, Pennsylvania, and Florida. And as with *Slim Forever,* a person who's never been to a Lean Line meeting can follow the program.

I always wondered what cybernetics meant and I was always too lazy to look it up in the dictionary, but the authors give us this definition: "a method which enables the human being to overcome seemingly impossible obstacles in order to reach desired goals." (That's the perfect definition of dieting!)

The cybernetics outlined here consist of a calorie-counting diet balanced with a behavior-modification program that is described in detail later, in Chapter 4. The Lean Line Diet has three elements:

1. The Basic Diet causes you to lose weight.
2. The Cruise Diet "prepares you psychologically for the time when you will need to maintain your weight loss, and provides easy-to-reach, short-term goals."
3. The Permanent Maintenance Plan "gives you a practical, easy-to-follow maintenance plan based on the nutritionally and psychologically sound principles you will have learned in the Basic and Cruise Diets."

There are all sorts of lists of allowed foods but the diet is easy to figure out. And you don't have to suffer from self-denial forever. The diet allows you to have half a doughnut or one and a half cups of popcorn or various other goodies—though only in precisely measured amounts, and only once a day.

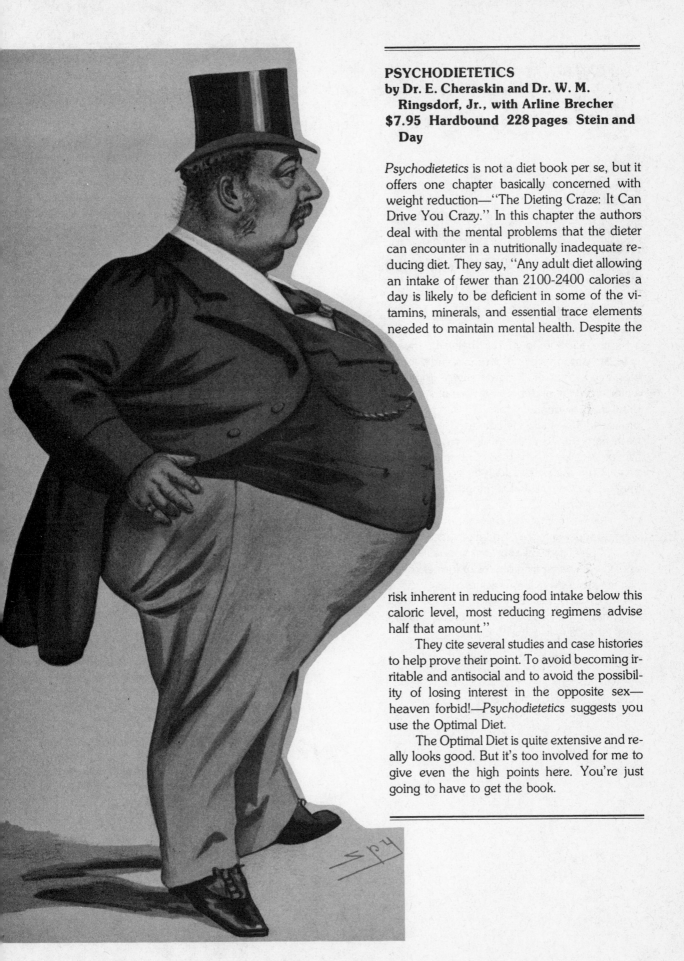

PSYCHODIETETICS
by Dr. E. Cheraskin and Dr. W. M. Ringsdorf, Jr., with Arline Brecher
$7.95 Hardbound 228 pages Stein and Day

Psychodietetics is not a diet book per se, but it offers one chapter basically concerned with weight reduction—"The Dieting Craze: It Can Drive You Crazy." In this chapter the authors deal with the mental problems that the dieter can encounter in a nutritionally inadequate reducing diet. They say, "Any adult diet allowing an intake of fewer than 2100-2400 calories a day is likely to be deficient in some of the vitamins, minerals, and essential trace elements needed to maintain mental health. Despite the risk inherent in reducing food intake below this caloric level, most reducing regimens advise half that amount."

They cite several studies and case histories to help prove their point. To avoid becoming irritable and antisocial and to avoid the possibility of losing interest in the opposite sex—heaven forbid!—*Psychodietetics* suggests you use the Optimal Diet.

The Optimal Diet is quite extensive and really looks good. But it's too involved for me to give even the high points here. You're just going to have to get the book.

YOU CAN BE FAT-FREE FOREVER
by Dr. L. Melvin Elting and Dr. Seymour Isenberg
$1.95 Paperback 218 pages Penguin Books

This is a weight-reduction book not a diet book. The authors, two New Jersey physicians specializing in weight control, do not like the word diet. They lay it right on the line on page 5: "In fact, obesity is not only a disease, it is a chronic, recurrent disease. It is incurable (although it may be controllable)." You can't get any plainer than that.

The authors call their weight-control method "The Food Intake Plan," and it's only one page long. The system has three parts: 1. You are allowed to nibble, between meals, specified amounts of certain fruits and vegetables; 2. you must drink eight 8-ounce glasses of water each day and three portions of specified dried fruits or cranberry jelly; 3. You may have protein foods—these include beef, lamb, veal, fresh ham, fish, and seafood, but no smoked fish or meats—in small amounts as often as needed. As the doctors tell you on their Food Intake Plan Sheet, "If it is not printed here do not eat or drink it."

This is a comprehensive diet book (sorry, weight-reduction book), and it includes discussions of most medical questions you're liable to ask. There are startling photos of former obese patients, and even some recipes.

There is one small problem with the book, and that's the cover—"before" and "after" shots of a cutie in a bikini. Ugh.

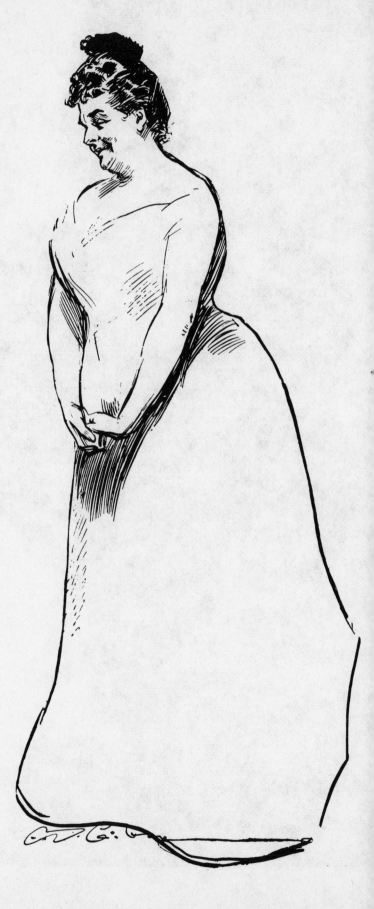

SLIM FOREVER: THE DIET CONTROL CENTER'S DIET
by Mary Sargent
$1.50 Paperback 215 pages Bantam Books

This book details the Diet Control Center's diet plan for their members. Diet Control Centers are diet groups in New York, New Jersey, Pennsylvania, Ohio, Florida, Wisconsin, and California, and their diet resulted from the work of three women who started experimenting with the proven, medically sound New York Health Department diet in an effort to add variety and ethnic foods to the menu.

The diet itself has a lot of protein—complete proteins that are found in meat, poultry, fish, cheese, eggs, and milk. And there is no calorie-counting, so you can put your socks on. You won't need your toes to help count.

Let's take a quick peek at the diet:

1. Three times a day, seven days a week, you must eat a specified amount of fish, poultry, veal, liver or other organ meats, cheese, or eggs.
2. Twice every day you are to have skim milk and related dairy products.
3. Twice every day, more often if you like, you are to choose from among a listing of required vegetables.
4. Every day you are required to eat certain fruits. The amount depends on your sex and age.
5. You are allowed to eat a specified amount of bread or equivalent food every day.

There are other required foods and optional foods, and a novel plus: you can have three alcoholic drinks a week, but only one drink on any given day. (Gotcha—you thought you could have three shooters in five minutes.) But there's nothing worse than a drunk dieter; they can be very mean.

Slim Forever is full of menus and gives you a number of recipes to choose from—which should help protect you from the monotony that is the greatest cause of diet failures.

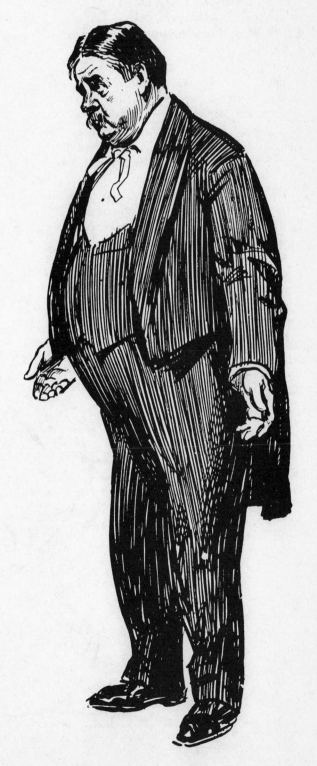

Carbohydrates, Protein, Fats, Fiber, Fructose, Etc.

DR. ATKINS' DIET REVOLUTION
by Robert C. Atkins, M.D.
$1.95 Paperback 324 pages Bantam Books

Whether or not Dr. Atkins' Diet is really a Revolution, there can be no denying that, with over three million copies of this book in print, Dr. Atkins has certainly reached a tremendous number of people. His diet is based on avoidance of foods containing carbohydrates—that is, fruits, vegetables, and grains.

The first week of the diet you are to eat no carbohydrates. You may eat all the protein and fat that you wish. You can stuff yourself with almost any type of meat, fish, or poultry. You can have green salads with the oiliest, most caloric dressing you can find—even Roquefort. For snacks you can eat cheese, pork rinds, deviled eggs, or any number of other goodies.

The dessert list—*list?*—the first week is limited to carbohydrate-free gelatin. The following weeks you can eat such things as mocha pie, cheesecake, and strawberries in artificially sweetened whipped cream, and you can top a meal off with heavy cream in your coffee. At breakfast, you can eat yourself into oblivion with eggs, ham, bacon, steak, and omelets.

All this is pretty straightforward; but then we come to Dr. Atkins' ace in the hole—ketones. According to Dr. Atkins, ketones are "little carbon fragments that are by-products of the incomplete burning of fat." As long as your body is excreting ketones, he says, your body is burning up fat. The way to find out if you're burning up your fat is by checking your urine daily with Ketostix. If the Ketostix turn purple, you know you are still burning up fat.

After the first week, there are four levels to your diet. With each level, you may add more foods with carbohydrates. But remember, your Ketostix must keep turning purple until you get down to the weight you want to reach. When you get there, you should be at your Critical Carbohydrate Level, which varies with the individual and also varies at different times of your life.

Almost 100 pages of the book are devoted to recipes and meal plans. Listen to the titles of

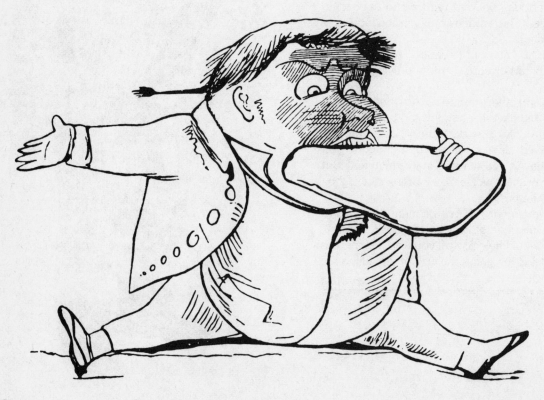

some of the recipes: Chicken Cordon Bleu, Shrimp and Lobster Cantonese, Hollandaise Sauce, and Coffee Walnut Chocolate Roll. It all sounds remarkable. But is it medically safe?

To help you make this decision, you might want to look at a statement published in 1973 by the American Medical Association's Council on Foods and Nutrition, entitled "A Critique of Low-Carbohydrate Ketogenic Weight Reduction Regimens. A Review of Dr. Atkins' Diet Revolution." And on April 12, 1973, Dr. Atkins testified before the Select Committee on Nutrition and Human Needs about his book and diet. His statement to the committee is printed on page 299 of *Dr. Atkins' Diet Revolution.* And on page 130, Dr. Atkins tells us: "Before any patient starts with me, I take a comprehensive series of blood tests, which I recommend you have your own physician give you, particularly if you have more than twenty pounds to lose." The decision, it seems, is up to you.

THE DOCTOR'S QUICK WEIGHT LOSS DIET
by Irwin Maxwell Stillman, M.D., and Samm Sinclair Baker
$1.25 Paperback 252 pages Dell Books

What can anyone say about a diet book that's sold five million copies? The diet must work, at least for a while, or a lot of folks are drinking an awful lot of water for nothing.

The Quick Weight Loss Diet is simple: basically it's a high-protein, low-fat, low-carbohydrate regimen, but it has its own special twist. You can eat all the lean beef, lamb, veal, chicken, turkey, fish, seafood, low-fat cottage cheese, and other skim milk cheeses you want. But—here's the twist—you must drink eight 10-ounce glasses of water every day. This quantity of water is in addition to whatever other liquids you drink during the day. According to Dr. Stillman, the water is needed to wash out all the "waste products or ashes of burnt fat."

The book also gives you sixty other "Quick Weight Loss" diets to choose from, plus a lot of diet tips. If you do go on the diet—which I like to call "The Big Flusher"—you'd better be on a first-name basis with your plumber.

THE DOCTOR'S QUICK INCHES-OFF DIET
by Irwin Maxwell Stillman, M.D., and Samm Sinclair Baker
$1.25 Paperback 310 pages Dell Books

The Diet Duo are at it again, but this time they're telling you how to lose inches instead of pounds. To do this, Dr. Stillman says, you should eat a low-protein diet of certain fruits, vegetables, soups, and—in small amounts—cereals, breads, crackers, and cookies. Plus you can have "very small" portions of such non-dietetic things as spaghetti, popcorn, or tapioca. You cannot eat such foods as meats, poultry, seafood, eggs, and cheese, all of which makes the Inches-Off Diet basically a vegetarian diet.

As in the original Stillman diet, you are to drink eight to ten cups or glasses of tea, coffee, diet soda, or water a day, but you add a vitamin-mineral pill every day. And since you don't have to avoid carbohydrates on this diet, you may also have one cocktail or glass of wine a day. So take a straight shot of booze, plant yourself a vegetable garden, and watch those inches fall off.

DR. STILLMAN'S 14-DAY SHAPE-UP PROGRAM
by Irwin Maxwell Stillman, M.D., and Samm Sinclair Baker
$1.75 Paperback 225 pages Dell Books

This book, published in 1974, was the late Dr. Stillman's last diet book. In the 14-Day Shape-Up Program, his diet is called the "Protein-Plus" Diet, but it's fundamentally unchanged from his original diet. The "Plus" with the "Protein" is a small amount of carbohydrates. You can eat "satisfying portions" of chicken, turkey, certain fish, certain seafood, meat with all the fat trimmed off, eggs (one or two at a time), certain vegetables including cauliflower, zucchini, and many others, specified cheeses, skim milk, yogurt, and a very small amount of bread or cake. You must drink at least ten glasses of permitted beverages a day, and you may have one cocktail a day. As with his other diets, there is no calorie-counting. The "Shape-Up Program" of the title is justified by a section at the end of the book outlining a stretching, bending, and walking routine.

I, for one, am going to miss Dr. Stillman on the Johnny Carson, Mike Douglas, Merv Griffin, and other talk shows. He sure was a distinct personality. He was very bright and a great and funny guest. But I could never figure out whether people were laughing with him or at him.

DR. SIEGAL'S NATURAL FIBER PERMANENT WEIGHT-LOSS DIET
by Sanford Siegal, D.O., M.D.
$1.75 Paperback 299 pages Dell Books

This is one complicated diet book. There are charts galore, recipes, and enough abbreviations to confuse the Signal Corps, so be prepared for some heavy concentration. The basic premise of the book, backed up by much research, is that we, you and I, do not eat enough natural fiber—we're not getting enough roughage in our meals, and since it therefore takes too long for us to evacuate our bowels, we are building up too many harmful bacteria and poisons in our systems. If we added natural fiber to our diets and made a few other simple changes in our eating habits, we could lose weight.

With the high-fiber diet you eat a minimum of ten to twelve grams of fiber every day and cut out all refined carbohydrates. You can do this by adding several tablespoons of bran to each meal (or by eating other foods with a high fiber content) and by staying away from refined sugar and flour. The book has a number of charts to help you determine the fiber content of many foods, and it also gives recipes to which you can add bran.

I must warn you that, to my taste buds, eating bran is not like eating hot roasted peanuts. Bran has to be disguised. But Dr. Siegal's book is so convincing in its advocacy of bran that you may find yourself running to your nearest store for a 100-pound bag of it.

THE SAVE YOUR LIFE DIET
by Dr. David Reuben, M.D.
$1.95 Paperback 172 pages
Ballantine Books

This is not primarily a weight-reducing diet book: it's Dr. Reuben's way of saying that we must add fiber to our diet to get our digestive systems functioning normally.

As Dr. Reuben puts it, "The basic principle of this reducing diet is to normalize the functioning of the digestive system—not to derange it as most other weight-reduction diets do." We can do this, he says, by adding roughage to our diet. This is what the doctor prescribes:

Cut out all low-roughage foods. Eat high-roughage foods. Eat moderate amounts of meat, fish, and poultry, and moderate amounts of fats and oils. Eat only whole grain bread and other whole grain flour products. Have no refined sugar and no alcoholic beverages. Eat raw fruits and vegetables, if possible. And add unprocessed miller's bran to the diet every day.

THE MIRACLE NUTRIENT
by Carl I. Flath
$1.95 Paperback 192 pages Bantam Books

The miracle nutrient here is the natural fiber found in grains—oatmeal, wheat, bran, and brown rice—as well as in raw fruits and vegetables, especially in the cellulose parts that we frequently throw away or that are lost in modern food processing. According to Mr. Flath, just half an ounce of fiber added to the daily diet can end or prevent constipation and other lower colonic disorders, cholesterol problems, appendicitis, varicose veins, diverticular disease, cardiovascular ailments, and even cancer of the colon and rectum.

The author also talks about the role fiber plays in nutrition, and offers easy exercises, dietary tips, and recipes on how to add the "miracle nutrient" to your diet.

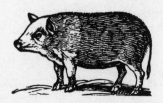

CARLTON FREDERICKS' HIGH-FIBER WAY TO TOTAL HEALTH
by Carlton Fredericks, Ph.D.
$1.95 Paperback 208 pages Pocket Books

Carlton Fredericks in this book extols the glories of the high-fiber diet. Besides blaming modern ills on our overprocessed food, from which vitamins, minerals, and roughage have been removed, Dr. Fredericks discusses the proper diets for digestive disorders, important differences in bran, ideal levels of fiber intake, and, most important, when to seek medical advice.

There are two chapters on how to lose weight on a high-fiber diet. The first details a substitution diet (no calorie-counting) in which you choose what to eat from lists of various low-calorie foods, adding one or two teaspoons of bran three times a day or taking two to four bran tablets with each meal, as well as taking a daily vitamin and mineral supplement.

The second diet is a high-fiber, low-carbohydrate reducing diet—which may sound like a contradiction since bran and fiber are rich in carbohydrates. But Carlton Fredericks stresses the unprocessed carbohydrates which are fiber sources: salads, raw fruits and vegetables, and a bran supplement. There are only six grams of carbohydrate in each tablespoon of bran, so you can take the full amount of bran you need and not go over your carbohydrate limit. All this is supposed to come to you in the form of six small meals a day, plus a vitamin and mineral supplement.

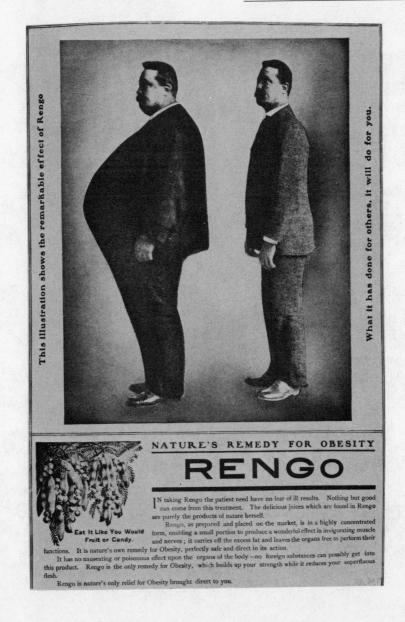

This illustration shows the remarkable effect of Rengo

What it has done for others, it will do for you.

NATURE'S REMEDY FOR OBESITY

RENGO

Eat It Like You Would Fruit or Candy.

IN taking Rengo the patient need have no fear of ill results. Nothing but good can come from this treatment. The delicious juices which are found in Rengo are purely the products of nature herself.

Rengo, as prepared and placed on the market, is in a highly concentrated form, enabling a small portion to produce a wonderful effect in invigorating muscle and nerves ; it carries off the excess fat and leaves the organs free to perform their functions. It is nature's own remedy for Obesity, perfectly safe and direct in its action.

It has no nauseating or poisonous effect upon the organs of the body—no foreign substances can possibly get into this product. Rengo is the only remedy for Obesity, which builds up your strength while it reduces your superfluous flesh.

Rengo is nature's only relief for Obesity brought direct to you.

DR. CARLTON FREDERICKS' LOW-CARBOHYDRATE DIET
by Carlton Fredericks, Ph.D.
$1.50 Paperback 188 pages Award Books

This is Carlton Fredericks' contribution to the low-carbohydrate diet field. Dr. Fredericks wrote this book before Dr. Atkins (see p. 12) wrote his; as Dr. Atkins' is more widely known, it must be that Dr. Atkins packaged his book better for the low-carbohydrate diet world.

Dr. Fredericks' system is to eat six small meals a day, each low in starch and sugar, high in protein, and moderately high in fat (about a fifth of this fat should be polyunsaturated to help in the burning of body fat). There is no counting of calories. The secret ingredient here is Vitamin C, taken orally as a mild diuretic. The book contains charts of the carbohydrate values of various foods, two food plans with seven days of menus, and some advice on how to stay down in weight, once you're there.

LOSE POUNDS THE LOW-CARBOHYDRATE WAY
by Myra Waldo
$1.25 Paperback 127 pages Signet Books

This diet is a low-carbohydrate diet like Dr. Atkins'. You must restrict your carbohydrate intake to sixty grams per day. But Ms. Waldo says that if you really want to peel off the pounds, cut the carbohydrates even further—though without falling below a minimum of 35

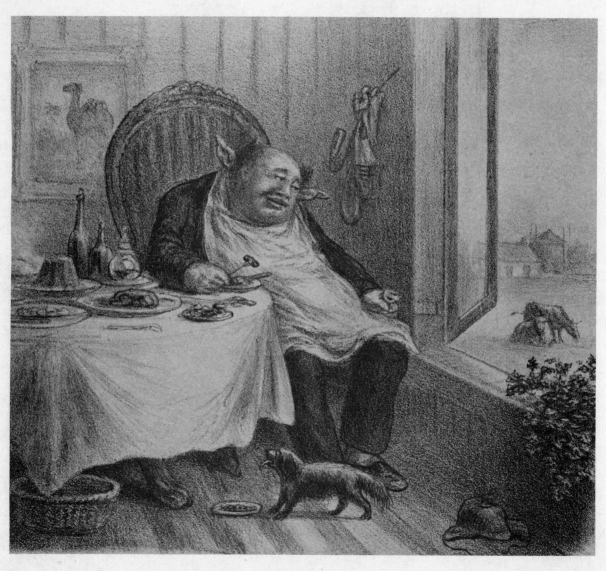

grams of carbohydrates per day. As a food and restaurant critic, Myra Waldo truly cares about what she puts into her mouth, so the menus (enough for seven days) and recipes feature juicy thick steaks, lobster dripping with butter sauce, salads loaded with mayonnaise, egg-plant caviar, ham-cheese soufflé, seafood New-burg, and cheese-stuffed crêpes. Carbohydrate counts for 2000 foods are also included. I am still in despair from having discovered that an average slice of watermelon has 58 grams of carbohydrate. What am I to do on those hot summer days when my teeth long to sink into a huge chunk of ice cold watermelon? Woe is me.

SECRETS FOR STAYING SLIM
by Lelord Kordel
$1.25 Paperback 176 pages Signet Books

With *Secrets for Staying Slim* you don't count calories, but you do eat (or drink):

1. Foods high in protein and low in animal fats and carbohydrates (there are lists, with al-lowable substitutions).
2. Liver twice a week and seafood four or five times a week.
3. Limited fresh fruits and fruit juices.
4. Only sixty grams of carbohydrates a day.
5. Lots of leafy greens and raw vegetables.
6. Lots of specified herbs, spices, seeds, and sauces.
7. All you want of unsweetened teas, coffees, clam juice, club soda, consommé, and bouillon.

In addition, three times a day around a half hour before eating, you're supposed to drink a combination of honey, safflower oil and cider vinegar.

Mr. Kordel also tells you about "crash" diets, fasting, and diets from Italy, Scandinavia, and Russia, and gives you a hot little chapter on "Obesity and Your Sex Life."

The last forty-four pages are devoted to such slimming recipes as Rabbit-Patch Salad, Stuffed Veal Birds, and Pineapple-Mint Frappé. The author's concoction of honey, safflower oil, and cider vinegar is called HOV (Hated Overweight Vanishes). I haven't tried it yet.

THE NEW CARBO-CAL WAY TO LOSE WEIGHT AND STAY SLIM
MARTINIS & WHIPPED CREAM
By Sidney Petrie with Robert B. Stone
95¢ Paperback 266 pages Paperback Library

Right off the bat, if you're like me and never chug-a-lugged a martini, or squirted whipped cream on top, you can still lose weight on this diet.

Now that I've straightened you out on one vital point, I can tell you that Mr. Petrie has devised a low-carbohydrate diet in which you count Carbo-Cals—units of measurement based on the fact that one gram of carbohydrate burns four calories. For instance, one small apple has 44 Carbo-Cals. You are to eat 250 Carbo-Cals per day. According to the author, you can eat fried foods, appetizers, gravies, sauces, dressings, ice cream, and, of course, martinis and whipped cream.

The book also has a list of 2500 foods with their Carbo-Cal counts, recipes, and information on how to shop wisely.

THE CARBO-CALORIE DIET
by Donald S. Mart
$1.50 Paperback 114 pages Dolphin Books

Eyeballs red from staring at the list of calorie-counts for the foods you eat? Tired of counting carbohydrates too? This book combines the two and offers a new angle for you to lose weight. You must use a formula to figure out the Carbo-Calories in the food you eat—but the book makes things easier by offering 106 pages of the Carbo-Calorie counts of various foods. Unless you eat exotic foods, you won't have to do much figuring.

Mr. Mart says that you should eat 100 Carbo-Calories per day to lose weight. At 100 Carbo-Calories per day, you are eating approximately 1200 calories and 60 grams of carbohydrates. But for good health you should not eat fewer than 58 Carbo-Calories per day. Some sample Carbo-Calorie counts from the book: one slice of pumpernickel bread has 16 Carbo-Calories; half a cup of creamed cottage cheese has 8; one chocolate-covered cherry has 15; and half a cantaloupe has 14.

SLIMMING DOWN
by Ed McMahon
$1.50 Paperback Warner Paperback
Library

Ed McMahon, as every tube-watcher knows, is Johnny Carson's pal with the great laugh on the *Tonight Show*. Over the years on the show, there's been a lot of kidding about Ed's weight—and, of course, his drinking. You could actually see how his weight went up and down on the show. But Ed's weight problem had started long before his days on television.

At birth Ed McMahon weighed nine pounds fourteen ounces. As he points out, that's a third more than the national average. After years of misery and dozens of futile diets, as he relates in *Slimming Down,* he came across *Martinis & Whipped Cream* by Sidney Petrie and Robert B. Stone (See p. 17), which "opened my eyes to a new way of getting rid of fat for good." He has built on this and added a few variations of his own, which he now shares with us.

In Ed's "Carbo-Cal" system, you try to limit yourself to 250 Carbo-Cals a day. To determine Carbo-Cal counts of the foods you want to eat, you can look at the list at the back of the book, and, for any foods not listed, you can use a formula which Ed provides. For example, it might interest you to know that one apple has 100 Carbo-Cals, while a bourbon and soda has none. (No wonder Big Ed likes this diet.)

Besides the Carbo-Cal tables and formula, there are sample menus, recipes, and Ed McMahon's own fat-fighting story. All written in a breezy, readable, enjoyable style.

DIET AWAY YOUR STRESS, TENSION & ANXIETY
THE FRUCTOSE DIET BOOK
by J. Daniel Palm, Ph.D.
$6.95 Hardbound 277 pages
Doubleday

The dust jacket of this book calls it: "A bold new diet that shows you how you can eat your way out of a number of disorders you may have eaten your way into in the first place.

Overeating, obesity, migraine headaches, alcoholism, schizophrenia, hypoglycemia, and hyperactivity—all may be controlled, by a program that pivots on the ingestion of fructose (fruit sugar)."

The author says that weight loss depends on using between 75 and 100 grams of fructose each day. The diet outlined is an exchange diet plan with seven groups of foods from which to choose. This way you may design your own diet program. There are also sample menus, recipes, and plenty of bar graphs and calorie charts.

Looking back at my own wonderful method of handling stress, tension, and anxiety, which was to stuff myself with goodies as quickly and fatteningly as possible, I find myself wondering if maybe this is a better way.

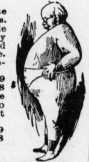
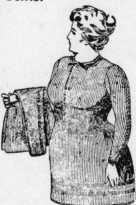

Special Diets

THE LOW FAT, LOW CHOLESTEROL DIET
by Clara-beth Young Bond, R.D.,
   E. Virginia Dobbin, R. D., Helen F.
   Gofman, M.D., Helen C. Jones, and
   Lenore Lyon
$8.95   Hardbound   512 pages
   Doubleday

With five authors collaborating, over 500 pages divided into thirty-two chapters, this book sets out to be (in the words of its publisher), "An authoritative and reliable guide to the planning and preparation of appetizing meals for any person whose doctor advises this diet for the prevention or treatment of heart diseases owing to hardening of the arteries."

Hundreds of recipes are included, all with a breakdown of the amounts of oil, cholesterol, saturated fat, linoleic acid, protein, carbohydrate, and calories each recipe contains, and there are chapters on how to change eating habits, what you should know about meat, and other useful—and basic—information. There is even a short course in nutritional science. Expensive, but worth it.

THE FAST-AND-EASY TEENAGE DIET
by Lois Lyons Lindauer
$1.25 Paperback 186 pages Award
   Books

Being a fat teenager is one of the saddest of fates. The teen years are a time of life when appearance is crucially important, and in this book the Director of The Diet Workshop (see Chapter 4) has addressed herself specifically to kids between the ages of twelve and twenty. She discusses the four basic foods all teenagers need, what you should eat and how much, and whether you need to diet at all. She tells how to kick the hamburger–French fries–soft drink habit, how to make slimming snacks and des-

serts, how to brown-bag a diet-conforming school lunch, and how to stay slim after the diet.

There are tips on handling a dinner date without revealing you're on a diet, what to do when you're trapped at a hotdog stand, ways to make up for "cheating" without starving yourself for days, and clothes and hair styles to make you look slimmer while you're losing weight.

If you're a chunky teenager, or know one, this book could be a great deal of help. Correcting bad eating habits early can save a lot of pain later in life.

THE DOCTOR'S QUICK TEENAGE DIET
by Irwin Maxwell Stillman, M.D., and
   Samm Sinclair Baker
$1.25 Paperback 254 pages Warner
   Paperback Library

Direct from the folks that gave you that five-million-copy best-seller, The Doctor's Quick Weight Loss Diet, there is now The Doctor's Quick Teenage Diet.

The QTD is an eat-all-you-want diet that consists of: one or two glasses of skim milk per day, lean meats, chicken, turkey, lean fish, seafood, eggs, cottage cheese, a daily vitamin-mineral tablet, beverages, and eight glasses of water per day.

Variations on this theme are developed: Super-Quick Teenage Diet, a 7-Day Quick Teenage Diet, several 7-Day Quick-Variety Diets, a Liquids-Only 1-Day Super-Quick Diet, and, for those who must have a little something extra, a Quick Teenage Dividend Diet.

There are also chapters on "Keep-Slim Eating for the Rest of Your Happier Life," recipes, questions and answers, and a "Memo to Parents: How to Help Your Teenager Slim Down and Keep Slim."

The cover of the book shows five teenagers eating pizza, soft drinks, and watermelon. If they can lose weight on that kind of diet, where was the good doctor when I weighed 240 pounds in the eighth grade?

"I think no virtue goes with size."
—Ralph Waldo Emerson

People say that all Americans are obsessed with diets, but for diabetics in particular a good diet is an absolute necessity. And a good source of diet information for diabetics is

"TOWARD GOOD CONTROL, A GUIDEBOOK FOR THE DIABETIC"
Ames Company
Division Miles Laboratories, Inc.
Elkhart, Indiana 46514

This booklet outlines a diet which has been worked out with the collaboration of the American Diabetes Association and the American Dietetic Association. Emphasizing the need for your doctor's cooperation and advice, the authors say, "Any of the meal plans your doctor prescribes for you may be coordinated with the Substitution System. In this system of six basic food Substitution Lists, an infinite variety of foods is available to make your menu interesting and still nutritionally adequate for your needs. The reason these six food categories are called Substitution Lists is because any food on each List can be substituted for any other food on that same List. You cannot go from one list to another in making substitutions."

Additional booklets on diets for diabetics available from the American Diabetes Association, Inc., 1 West 48th Street, New York, New York 10017 are:

"Meal Planning with Exchange Lists" and "A Cookbook for Diabetics"
"The Calculating Cook," by Jeanne Jones
"Diabetic Cooking Made Easy," by Virginia M. Donahue
"How Diabetics Can Eat Wisely," by Dorothy Tompkins Revell

All right, Americans, we eat too much. We average about 3200 calories a day. Only three countries top us in caloric intake.
They're Ireland, 3375; Argentina, 3360; and Denmark, 3255.
Don't start sticking out your chest. Remember that people in these countries are far more active physically than we are in America.

Manipulating Your Metabolism

METABOLICS
PUTTING YOUR FOOD ENERGY TO WORK
by Lawrence E. Lamb, M.D.
$9.95 Hardbound 264 pages Harper & Row

Heavy reading here, but you'll get an education. The author, who writes a daily health column that runs in more than 700 newspapers, believes that no one can grasp the secrets of good health or successful dieting without first knowing how the body uses food to release energy. He points out that every cell in the body is a chemical processing plant in which food, once eaten, is converted into simple chemicals by a process called metabolism. Hence the title of this book: *Metabolics*—the study of what the body does with food.

Dr. Lamb postulates that people gain weight when they consume an excessive number of calories while they are not doing anything to burn them up. Dr. Lamb calls these "overhead" calories and offers a method for counting them. He points out that as a person gets older his basal metabolism (the turnover of calories used by the body while at rest under normal conditions) decreases. So if a forty-year-old man continues to eat as much as he did at twenty, and exercises just as much and as hard, he will still get fat. The author includes a chart giving standards for calorie intake at different ages. Using this plus his method for counting "overhead" calories, along with a balanced diet, should keep you sleek with loads of energy.

THE DOCTORS' METABOLIC DIET
by William F. Kremer, M.D., and Laura Kremer, M.D.
$6.95 Hardbound 192 pages Crown

The Doctors Kremer treat every overweight person, regardless of age or sex, as an individual, which automatically makes this an unusual weight-reduction book. And the authors even spout a little heresy, pointing out that some people who are overweight may be better off as they are: "Happiness through thinness may be an illusion."

The premise of this book is that losing weight is not as simple as eating less and counting calories—each individual must have a diet geared to his own specifications. In support of this premise the authors include discussions of metabolism, eating habits and how to change them, and hunger and appetite and how to control them.

Beyond these generalities, the authors offer a specific diet system based on two new techniques that I've never seen in any other diet book or article:

1. The best way to diet is to eat no breakfast at all. Certain foods stimulate your appetite so that you eat all day long.
2. One day a week is a fast day, during which you eat a few nibbles of "chew food." Some of the chew foods are raw carrots, raw apples, raw cauliflower, and fresh raw pineapple.

A fasting day is observed only until you reach your desired weight. Then you can increase food intake by one-sixth without messing up your diet patterns.

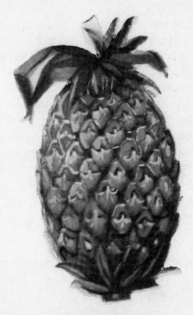

THE SEXY PINEAPPLE DIET
by Inge and Sten Hegeler
75¢ Paperback 124 pages Award Books

The authors are from Denmark; before taking on the heavies in the weight-reduction world, they wrote the best-selling *ABZ of Love*. Come to think of it, *The ABZ of Love* could be a diet book, too.

The Sexy Pineapple Diet consists of eating pineapple two days a week. That means pineapple only. The other five days you can eat what you want in moderation.

On the cover of the book it says if you stick to this diet, you will have greater sexual capacity. So I ran right out and bought the biggest pineapple I could find. It sure didn't look very sexy, and besides that it hurt me when I kissed it.

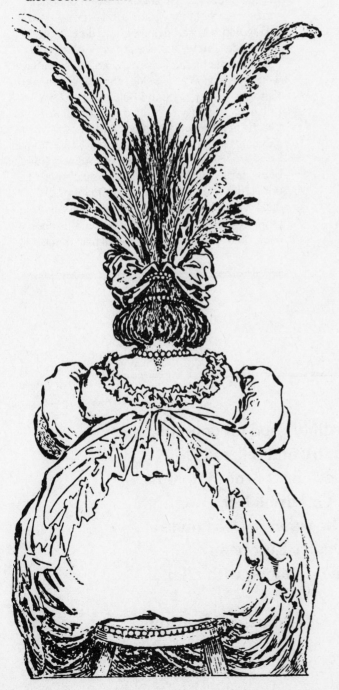

Fasting

THE LAST CHANCE DIET
by Dr. Robert Linn with Sandra Lee
 Stuart
$10.00 Hardbound 251 pages Lyle
 Stuart, Inc.

When all else has failed you may as well give up eating—or so say the authors of this grimly titled book.

In the Last Chance Diet you eat no solid food. What does pass your lips is a liquid formula, "composed of all the amino acids needed to form a protein molecule." Dr. Linn calls the formula Prolinn. Prolinn supplies the protein your body needs so that you won't use your lean body mass for energy. Only the useless fat disappears. In addition to Prolinn, you must take vitamin and mineral supplements, two to four grams a day of potassium, and higher levels of folic acid than are found in nonprescription multiple vitamins. Every day you must drink almost two quarts of liquids: water, coffee, tea, or sugarless soda.

FASTING: THE ULTIMATE DIET
by Allan Cott, M.D., with Jerome Agel
 and Eugene Boe
$1.75 Paperback 148 pages Bantam
 Books

After reading the first ten pages of this book, I wanted to rush right out and start fasting. And I'll bet you a stretch mark that if you read this book, you will too. I've never read a more persuasive diet book.

The author wisely says, "I cannot stress this too strongly: You should consult your doctor before beginning even a brief fast, just as you would before beginning any diet."

Once you've done that, Dr. Cott and his collaborators have devised a whole system for weight reduction and weight control. The book tells you how to fast (and how not to); it spells out how fasting works; it draws the line between people who should and those who shouldn't fast.

Whatever your problems, according to this book, fasting will straighten you out, whether you suffer from insomnia or a diminished sex drive. I'm not worried about my sex drive at the moment; I have a tough enough time just getting a date. But maybe fasting will help that too.

"Fasting can be incredibly good for you, too. When I'm in the country and relaxed, I go on juice fasts for a week or so—nothing but juice I make myself. Or I drink hot water for days at a time. The water in this country is terrible, though. I carry European bottled water with me . . . along with all my vitamin pills."

—Marisa Berenson

FASTING: THE SUPER DIET
by Shirley Ross
$1.75 Paperback 188 pages
Ballantine Books

For me, there's always been something fascinating about fasting. I tried it once and got to three in the afternoon before I couldn't take it any more and just had to eat. I flunked fasting. But stories about people who have gone in for fasting are so inspirational. They always make me want to stop eating immediately—I have visions of losing weight, cleaning out my system, and giving my poor body a rest.

This fasting book has that effect—it's a personal account of Shirley Ross's fasting regimens, beginning with the history of fasting from antiquity and culminating in the story of a fifty-seven-day fast. The book also explains what happens when you fast and what you should do if you are going to fast and even has a section on "fasting resorts."

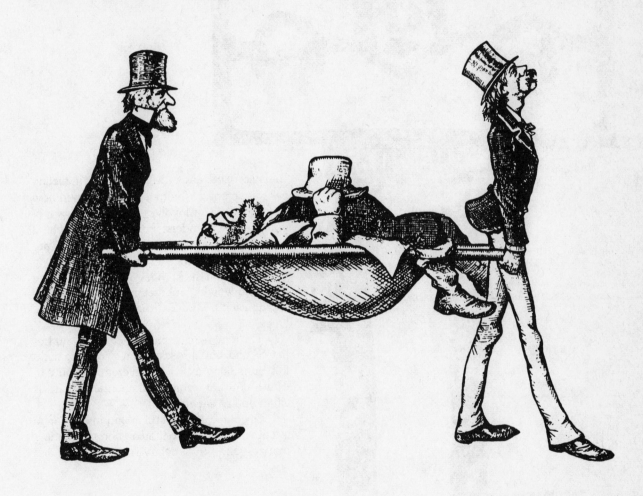

BEHAVIOR MODIFICATION

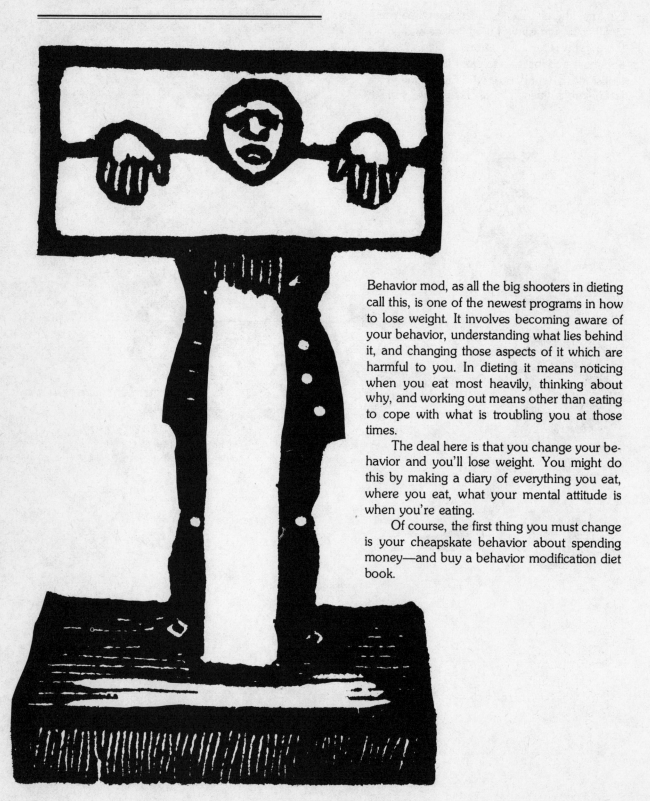

Behavior mod, as all the big shooters in dieting call this, is one of the newest programs in how to lose weight. It involves becoming aware of your behavior, understanding what lies behind it, and changing those aspects of it which are harmful to you. In dieting it means noticing when you eat most heavily, thinking about why, and working out means other than eating to cope with what is troubling you at those times.

The deal here is that you change your behavior and you'll lose weight. You might do this by making a diary of everything you eat, where you eat, what your mental attitude is when you're eating.

Of course, the first thing you must change is your cheapskate behavior about spending money—and buy a behavior modification diet book.

PERMANENT WEIGHT CONTROL, A TOTAL SOLUTION TO THE DIETER'S DILEMMA
by Michael J. Mahoney, Ph.D., and Kathryn Mahoney, M.S.W., M.S.
$7.95 Hardbound 177 pages W.W. Norton

The two authors, clinical psychologists, say that the way to lose weight and keep it off is to change your behavior of eating. And the way to do that is to start asking yourself some questions: How fast do you eat? Where do you eat? What do you think about when you eat? Do you eat when you are tense?

You have to be your own personal scientist. The authors show you how to gather information about your eating habits and attitudes, and how to discover the hidden patterns in this behavior. Then they give you strategies for self-control—a step-by-step program with such relaxation exercises as eating with your left hand to slow you down. (I'm going to try that myself.) The idea behind all this is that after you understand what makes you think and act as you do about food, then you can make the kind of basic changes that will help you lose weight and keep if off permanently.

This is not really a diet book with lists of forbidden foods and a prescribed food program—it's an exercise book for your body from the eyebrows up.

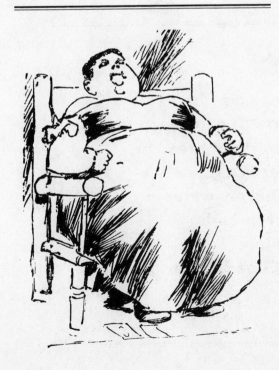

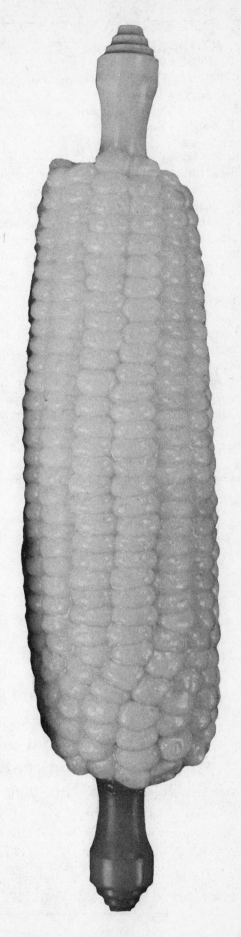

HOW TO BE A WINNER AT THE WEIGHT LOSS GAME
by Walter H. Fanburg, M.D., and Bernard M. Snyder, M.D.
$1.50 Paperback 128 pages
Ballantine Books

Another book that focuses on how you eat—where, why, how much, how fast, and under what emotional conditions. The authors are psychiatrists who specialize in the treatment of obesity using the principles of behavior modification. Their program begins with a detailed record of seven days of your eating life: you must write down everything you eat, and record the reasons for which, and conditions under which, you're eating. You evaluate the results, and then through the use of self-help charts, exercises, and sample menus, evolve a weight-loss curriculum tailor-made for your purposes.

Also included are tips on eating at the proper speed to lose weight (*don't* gobble your food), choosing your own special dining area, and gauging other people's effect on your eating.

THE FREEDOM DIET: *GAMES DIETERS PLAY*
by Leslie Jane Maynard
$8.95 Hardbound 151 pages
Frederick Fell

Everyone likes games except me. While others are playing Monopoly and backgammon, I'm looking in the refrigerator.

In this diet book, Ms. Maynard, who lost ninety pounds, has discovered some games dieters play such as the "Continual Open-and-Shut the Refrigerator" Game, the "If Nobody Sees, It Doesn't Count" Game, the "I Have a Hurt and Have to Make It Better" Game, the "I'm Only Buying It For . . ." game, the "On-And-Off the Scale Hop" Game, and eleven other embarrassingly real dieting games every overweight person will recognize.

There are also chapters entitled "How to Eat around the World," the "International Buffet," and "How to Eat at Fast Food Restaurant Chains."

So if you're tired of eating Doritos as you play Scrabble, give this number a run through. The problem with the pudgy games you're playing is that the only winner is the Grim Reaper.

"For forty years I never had a weight problem, but I sure do now. (I can't see how anyone can survive without bread or pasta.) What works for me is a three-day fast. I don't eat a thing, just sip water or juice. That way I drop five pounds. Anyone else would lose ten."

—Gina Lollobrigida

THE PSYCHOLOGIST'S EAT ANYTHING DIET
by Leonard Pearson, M.D., and Lillian R. Pearson, M.S.W., with Karola Saekel
$1.75 Paperback 254 pages Popular Library

According to the authors of this book, there are "humming foods" and "beckoning foods." Humming foods are foods we think about, even yearn for, without seeing them ("Desire for the food comes from the inner depths. The food may not even be immediately available."), while beckoning foods weren't on our minds until we saw them, but are immediately available ("It looks good. You'd enjoy it, but you don't crave it."). It's no good trying to ignore humming foods, say the authors: "If you don't follow your craving, if you don't eat the food that hums and eat a beckoning food instead you will not feel satisfied."

 The whole book is full of sensuous exercises dealing with food such as The Beer Exercise, sipping it through a straw; The Peanut Exercise, rolling one peanut around in your mouth; The Chocolate Exercise, taking one chocolate kiss and messing around with it in your mouth. I was starving by the time I got through this section.

 In addition, the book is loaded with case histories, and it has a question-and-answer section at the end with the most ridiculous diet questions I've ever seen. One sample question: "I'm eating all the food I like most of the day, and I'm gaining weight. How do you explain that?" But admittedly, the questions do reflect real attitudes. Maybe the point is to get them down on paper and see how silly they are.

HOW TO SAVE YOUR LIFE
by Earl Ubell
$2.25 Paperback 308 pages Penguin Books

Earl Ubell believes that the only way to lose weight and keep it off is to change the behaviors that lead to overeating. So he's developed a step-by-step program to get your imagination under conscious control. Here's the way it works:

1. high-calorie-food picture in your mind;
2. unpleasant thought (should wipe out food image);
3. stop the thought (should wipe out unpleasant thought);
4. low-calorie-food picture in your mind;
5. pleasant thought (should replace or fuse with low-calorie-food image).

As you can tell from the title, the trigger for this behavior modification is fear. Here is one of the suggestions for an unpleasant thought: "A picture of yourself as a huge, obese person unable to escape from a sinking ship because you are so fat you cannot fit through the escape hatch." Then there's the pleasant thought: "A beach with the ocean rolling in, walking with someone you love." Now that's nice.

 Additional chapters deal with drugs, alcohol, cigarettes, and sex and behavior—which makes this somewhat more than a diet book.

THE ONLY DIET THAT WORKS
by Herbert Brean
75¢ Paperback 155 pages Award Books

No messing around with this book. Herb tells you right off that this is the only way to lose weight. He uses behavior modification and says there are no calorie charts, no overnight miracles, no psychoanalysis. Mr. Brean offers a self-help program that will change your behavior.

 For instance, *"Be Good To Yourself."* You must watch your food like crazy but see a play each week, buy a new hat or necktie, or have an extra drink once in a while. *"Get Mad"*: Get mad at the folks who have kidded you along with temporary changes in your eating habits. Get mad at the people who forced skimmed milk or bananas down your throat. *"Try New Ways of Eating"*: Change your food habits. Cut out the cream in coffee or try bouillon instead of coffee (with coffee at four bucks a pound as I write this, that's a great suggestion). Eliminate one small item every day and you won't notice the difference but you'll notice the difference in your body.

 There's also a fourteen-day diary to help you analyze your thoughts and feelings about your eating habits.

 So sharpen up your pencil and you'll sharpen up your build. I like the part about getting mad. Right this minute, GRRR, I'm so mad I could grind up a cherry pie with my bare teeth.

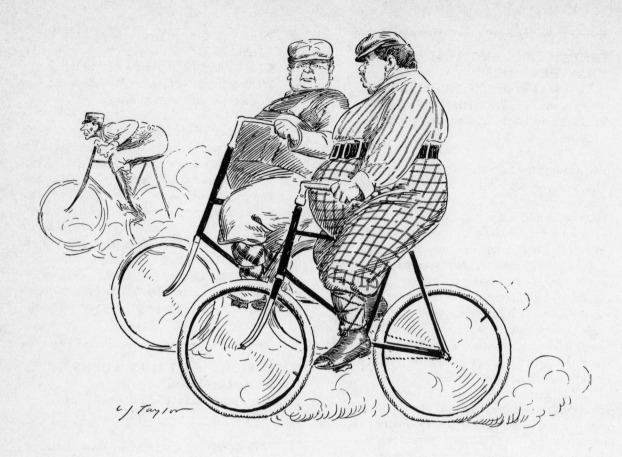

THE THIN BOOK BY A FORMERLY FAT
PSYCHIATRIST
by Theodore Isaac Rubin, M.D.
$1.25 Paperback 123 pages Pinnacle
Books

I read this diet book several years ago, and while rereading parts of it for this catalog, I have rediscovered many insights into obesity, such as the importance of routines and schedules, and how psychotherapy can affect dieting.

But I saw Dr. Rubin on a talk show several months ago, and he didn't look that thin to me. Which means that even diet-book authors must practice eternal vigilance, as we all must do, to stay thin. What a drag.

FAT FREE
COMMON SENSE FOR YOUNG WEIGHT
WATCHERS
by Sara Gilbert
$5.95 Paperback 114 pages Macmillan

A well-written, noncondescending book for overweight teenagers and their parents. Sara Gilbert proceeds from the premise that "When high school students are asked to list the medical and personal problems that bother them, concern about weight is the problem most frequently noted. Most important, excessive weight gain during adolescence can be a major cause of adult obesity."

The book discusses what overweight really is, "social" eating, behavior modification (with such chapters as "Is It All in Your Head?" and

"Making Up Your Mind"), and it has a no-non-sense prescriptive section on "What You Can Do About Fat." Also included are a calorie and carbohydrate chart, and resource listings of where you can find out more about teenage obesity.

This is an excellent primer for the over-weight adolescent. I only wish I could have read it as a teenager. (Knowing me, though, I probably would have read it while eating a dozen glazed doughnuts.)

ONE BOWL
by Don Gerrard
$1.45 Paperback 55 pages
Bookworks Books

This is a slim little volume that has an underground following—a countercultural diet book that might easily be subtitled "The Inner Game of Weight Control."

According to the author, who lost twenty pounds in eight weeks, "You gain weight because your head makes food decisions that ignore what your body wants." If you listen to your internal sounds without external noise, if you look at your whole person instead of at your stomach, you will change your eating habits.

The way to do this, explains the author, is to choose a bowl out of which you will eat all your food; then eat in courses and eat alone.

There is much more to the book than can be conveyed here, and the theories behind the one-bowl system are fascinating and somewhat mystical. So read the book, go out to your local dime store or museum, drop a quarter or a couple of grand for a Ming Dynasty Bowl of your choice, and lose weight.

EAT AND RUN
YOUR 1977 DIET, EXERCISE & ENGAGEMENT CALENDAR
by Jan Ferris Koltun
$4.95 Paperback unpaged Holt, Rinehart and Winston

The logical extension of the self-help records and charts in behavior-modification diet books, this is a spiral calendar for 1977 in which you record all meals and snacks—what you eat, when, and where, as well as how many calories you consume—exercise, engagements, and comments for each day of the year. This way you can keep watch on yourself and plan ahead at the same time: for instance, if you have a heavy social week coming up, you can arrange your diet accordingly.

As the author says, "Written evidence can help motivate you to take responsibility for your body." Working with the dieticians at Boston's Peter Bent Brigham Hospital, she developed three basic steps for reorganizing your diet:

1. "You need to be aware and in control of your food intake."
2. "You must evaluate the nutritional content of what you eat."
3. "You need to modify your eating to meet your new goals."

This calendar, she and her collaborators say, "will give you self-documented feedback and a realistic view of what has happened to you in the previous year." The calendar also features exercises, nutritional information, cartoons, aerobics, different diets, recipes for such things as make-it-yourself yogurt and steamed vegetables, exercise-calorie equivalents, and other goodies.

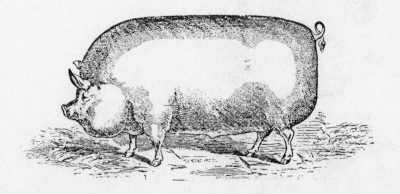

GETTING FIT AND KEEPING FIT

Hey, pals, I'm not going to kid you. We all know that getting in shape and staying there takes a little work, sweat, and discipline. You have to pay for your new bod.

Since I'm not hot on any of the above, I just sit in my recliner and dream about being a new man. I'm what you'd call an armchair exerciser. I read everything I can about exercise and even occasionally try it for a week or so. I buy all the latest equipment, give it a couple of grunts and slide it right in the closet behind my old fraternity sweat shirt. I probably have more stuff in there than Wilson Sporting Goods has in their warehouse.

What we have in this section are some of the tools and methods to tighten up saggy muscles, put sparkle in those beautiful eyes, and more spring in those flat feet.

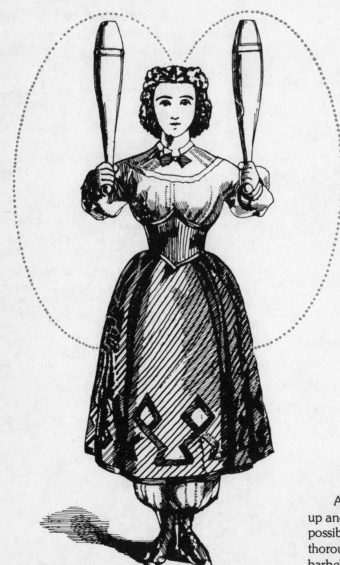

As for me, I'll keep walking and running up and down stairs to keep in shape. You can't possibly be as lazy as I am, so give this section a thorough going over. You could find the magic barbell.

THE BARBELL WAY TO PHYSICAL FITNESS
by Bruce Randall
Foreward by Stan Musial
$7.95 Hardbound 147 pages
Doubleday

When I was a chubby teenager (remember, I weighed 240 pounds in the eighth grade), every guy I knew lifted weights. Some lasted a week; others went straight through college grunting and groaning. As for me, I had a great time watching them work out and laughing over my bags of goodies. The only bar I ever wanted to press was a frozen Snickers—to my bosom.

Weight-training does work, if you work. Bruce Randall (Mr. Universe) has written a very readable, easy-to-follow weight-lifting book for beginners. But the beginners can be anyone from executives to housewives to growing children. There are over 190 photographs that accompany the text. Everything is explained in great detail. And he answers almost every question you might have.

There is one chapter on diet. Mr. Randall emphasizes that *protein* is what builds muscles, exercise *develops* them. If you've decided to "pump iron" and develop those "lats, pecs, and delts," this is an excellent book to start.

SLIMMING WITH WEIGHTS: A WOMAN'S GUIDE TO FIGURE CONTROL AND STRENGTH POTENTIAL
Text and photographs by Ingrid Schultheis
$8.95 Hardbound San Francisco Book Company

Women needn't be afraid of bulging muscles, according to this book, which outlines a three-times-a-week program for losing weight, trimming muscles, taking off inches, and increasing strength.

You can get the equipment at department and sporting goods stores, or you can make it at home at no cost. Each exercise is shown in step-by-step photographs.

I'll tell you this much. If I take out a woman and find that she's lifting weights, I'm not going to mess around with her unless she says it's okay.

According to the Metropolitan Life Insurance Co., 12% of men and women between the ages of twenty and twenty nine are more than 20% overweight. That means if you're supposed to weigh 150 pounds, you weigh at least 180 pounds.

In the thirty to thirty nine age group, 25% of American women are more than 20% overweight; from forty to forty nine, the figure is 40% and from fifty to fifty nine, exactly 46% are more than 20% too heavy.

Men aren't so overweight. From thirty to thirty nine, the rate is 25%, the same as women; from 40 to 49 the figure is 32% and 34% between the ages of fifty and fifty nine.

ROYAL CANADIAN AIR FORCE EXERCISE PLANS FOR PHYSICAL FITNESS
$1.75 Paperback 175 pages Pocket Books

Anyone who has ever thrown himself down on the floor and grunted through a couple of push-ups before quitting, exhausted, must have heard of the Royal Canadian Air Force Exercise Plan.

There are two basic plans in this book. One is called 5BX—an eleven-minute-a-day plan for men—and the other is called XBX—a twelve-minute-a-day plan for women. The time limit for each exercise plan remains the same throughout, but the number of times for each exercise and difficulty are increased as you progress.

The RCAF Plan was developed after World War II. It took two years of research by a team of doctors, scientists, and physical education specialists to devise the program of five basic exercises for men and ten basic exercises for women. The program was also devised for people of any age or physical condition to achieve and maintain desirable levels of physical fitness.

As for weight control, they suggest you see your doctor before starting any diet. But as they say, "Research has shown clearly that the most effective way of taking off weight and keeping it off is through a program which combines exercise and diet."

THE COMPLETE ILLUSTRATED BOOK OF YOGA
by Swami Vishnudevananda
$1.95 Paperback 411 pages Pocket Books

Every morning when I get up, I do a five-minute shoulder stand, which is a yoga posture. I do this to save my hair and make me smarter, since according to what I've read, the blood rushing to your head enriches the scalp and brain. Therefore I should have stopped losing my hair and become the shrewdest businessman in the Western Hemisphere. None of this has come true so far, but who knows? Friends who are yoga enthusiasts swear by it. And the things they can do with their bodies would make a pretzel hurt.

Anyway, this is a book of complete yoga training, with 146 photographs of the Swami doing all the postures. According to the book, yoga can do everything from reducing excess fat to banishing constipation.

As for diet, the Swami suggests that you fast once a week, drinking only water. Eventually, he says, you should become a total vegetarian.

I would check with my doctor before doing any of this unless you walk into your doctor's office and find him relaxing on a bed of nails.

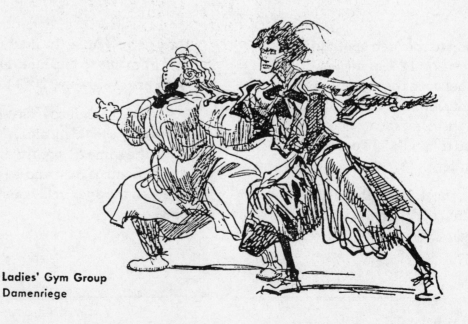

Ladies' Gym Group
Damenriege

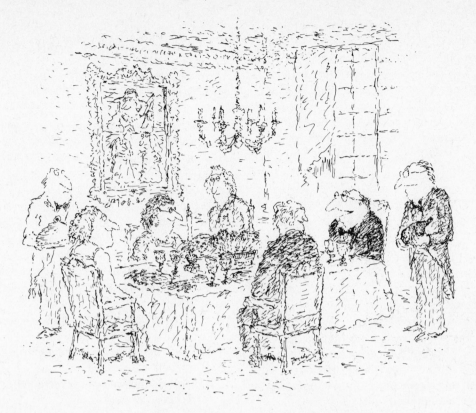

"While I rather enjoy pistachio, almond fudge, and English-toffee twirl, I think my very favorite is still plain vanilla with sprinkles."

HOW TO KEEP SLENDER AND FIT AFTER THIRTY
by Bonnie Prudden
$1.75 Paperback 302 pages Pocket Books

There are a couple of chapters dealing with eating and diets in this book by veteran exercise guru Bonnie Prudden, but the main business is getting you in shape. There are chapters on testing yourself for physical fitness, trimming the figure, reducing tension through exercise, walking, and "Sexercise."

Don't worry, this book is not rated "X," and you don't have to bring it home in a plain brown wrapper. The "Sexercise" chapter is an honest and forthright discussion of eighteen different exercises which can improve your sex life, illustrated with photographs of Ms. Prudden (fully clothed and alone). And this is only one chapter in an excellent and thorough book. The other chapters cover exercises from isometrics to aerobics, and you can pick and choose to fit your individual needs. There are almost 300 how-to-do-it photographs.

TOTAL FITNESS IN 30 MINUTES A WEEK
by Laurence E. Morehouse, Ph.D., and Leonard Gross
$1.95 Paperback 255 pages Pocket Books

This entertaining and informative book was a smash best-seller last year. Dr. Laurence Morehouse helped keep the astronauts fit in space with an easy, relaxed, no-sweat routine that you can follow too: it involves only thirty minutes a week, and he says it can get us all back into shape. He doesn't get into the exercises themselves until page 211, when he explains the "Three Short Steps to Fitness": "One minute of limbering, four minutes of muscle building and five minutes of any continuous activity that raises your heart rate to the desired level." In the remainder of the book he gives you exercises for limbering, muscle building, and heartbeat; there is also a chapter entitled "How to Lose Weight Forever." Dr. Morehouse suggests a loss of one pound a week. In order to do this, you must burn up 3500 calories of fat or 500 calories per day. So you should cut out

200 calories of food and use 300 calories in physical activity.

The giving up of 200 calories is easy—you just have to cut out two cups of coffee with sugar and cream or twelve potato chips. But the exercise part could be tough. Dr. Morehouse says that, to use up only 100 calories, we have to run for seven minutes, play tennis for fourteen minutes, or take a shower for thirty-one minutes. Really.

YOGA FOR PHYSICAL FITNESS
by Richard L. Hittleman
$1.50 Paperback 255 pages Warner Paperback Library

Richard Hittleman is television's famous yoga instructor, and in this book he has combined step-by-step instructions with over 250 photos to give you one of the best introductions to yoga around. If I can follow the instructions, and get myself into a semblance of these yoga postures, you know how good the explanations must be.

You can choose from fifty-eight yoga techniques that he says will help you with weight control, improve your health, increase vitality, make you relax, and just generally make you feel good all over. And it only takes minutes a day.

JOGGING, AEROBICS, AND DIET
by Roy Ald
$1.25 Paperback 191 pages Signet Books

The best explanation of this book comes from its author: "This plan is as natural as breathing: aerobics is a method of expanded oxygen consumption within the body, and jogging is its most effective practice. Aerobic exercise, combined with a diet patterned on your individual needs, can win you improved appearance, weight and appetite control, and a less stressful, healthier life." Some of the exercises Mr. Ald suggests are the neck swivel, the shoulder roll, push-ups, the jogtrot, and plain and simple running.

In addition, there are three different diets:

1. The Fitness Diet for those who are up to 6 percent overweight.
2. The Reducing Diet for those who are 6 to 16 percent overweight.
3. The Reducing Diet, more strictly applied, for those who are 16 percent or more overweight.

There are recommended menus and recipes for many of the menu items.

This book takes careful reading, and a slide rule could be helpful in deciphering the many charts, abbreviations, and directions. Some of it was confusing, but then I confuse easily.

Between twenty-five and forty-five percent of the adults in this country are more than twenty percent overweight, according to recent United States Public Health surveys. In a world still plagued by problems of malnutrition and starvation, the major nutritional affliction in this country is obesity.

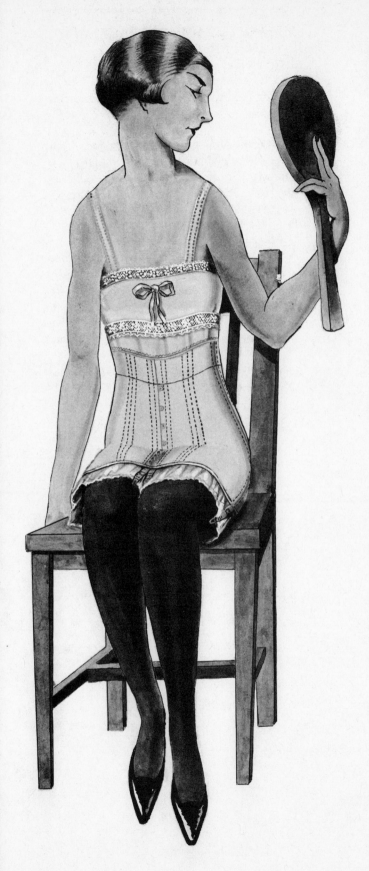

THE 14-DAY MIRACLE MAKE-OVER PROGRAM
by Zina Provendie
$1.50 Paperback 206 pages Award Books

Give yourself a couple of weeks and Zina Provendie promises to do a real job on you: for fourteen days you make over a different part of your body each day, until your whole body is transformed. For instance, the first day is "The Way You Wear Your Bones," the sixth day is "The Bath Ritual," and the eighth day is "Save the Face Day." Those are big orders for just twenty-four hours. The most important day for all of us is the second day, or "The 14-Day Slim-Down" (diets).

Ms. Provendie has included some interesting figure and diet information. She shows you how to use a Wrist Computer Chart to make allowances for your particular body peculiarities. There's a 1000-calorie Slim Down complete with menus and substitution lists so you won't get bored on the diet. Included, too, is the Prudent Diet by Dr. Norman Jolliffe, which Weight Watchers uses. And there are chapters on Spot Slim-Downs and Shape-Ups for such things as Dowager's Hump, Fatty Shoulder Pads, Saddlebags, Bottom, and Thighs.

THE CAREER GIRL'S DIET AND BEAUTY BOOK
by Joan Dunn
$1.25 Paperback 159 pages Award Books

This is a witty and easy-to-read survey of the diet and beauty field today by Joan Dunn, who writes the dieter's column for *Cosmopolitan* magazine. There are chapters on medical advice; diet plans for spring, summer, fall, and winter; exercises; recipes; helpful hints for dieters; Joan Dunn's personal dieting experiences; and a calorie list of common foods and their calories. The whole book is a grab bag of helpful weight-reduction information; even if you're not a career girl, you can learn something here.

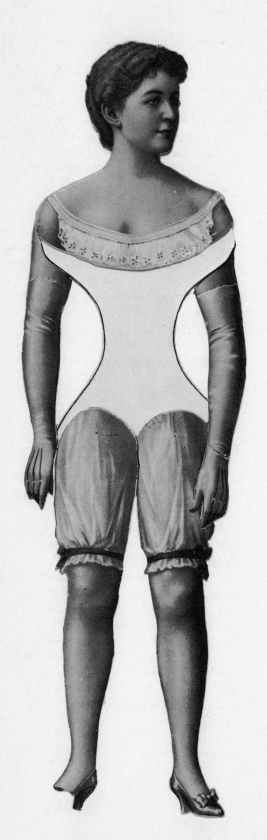

THE MODELS' WAY TO BEAUTY, SLENDERNESS & GLOWING HEALTH
by Oleda Baker with Bill Gale
$1.75 Paperback 213 pages Ballantine Books

Question: Who are the skinniest, most beautiful people in the world?

Answer: Those fashion models.

Q: How do they get and stay that thin and beautiful?

A. Read this book.

Q. Be more specific, big boy.

A. According to the author, the way to lose weight and keep it off is to choose a diet. Either a low-carbohydrate diet, a five-day diet, a high-protein diet, Gaylord Hauser's Ten-Day Diet, or the Adam and Eve Diet (you eat apples). Also become enthusiastic about your diet. Be a flamboyant calorie-counter, decorate your pantry, have a weigh-in, and keep a photo album of your progress.

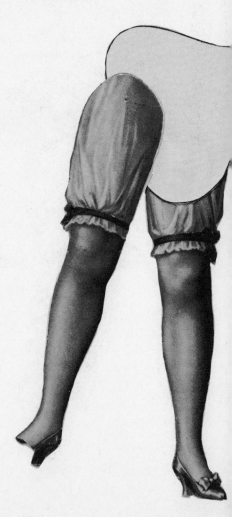

Q. All right, that takes care of the thin part. Now, how do I become beautiful?

A. Okay, Slim, there are chapters on "Glamour Vitamins," "Healthy Skin," "Healthy Hair," "Strong Eyes," "Sexy Teeth," and "Pretty Teeth."

Q. Terrific. Is there anything more about losing weight?

A. Yup. "How To Dine Out and Still Lose Weight," "How to Dress and Look Slimmer in Ten Minutes," and recipes for many low-calorie dishes. There's also slimming and beauty tips from top fashion models.

Q. When do I start looking like Candice Bergen?

A. Soon, very soon. And when it happens, give me a ring.

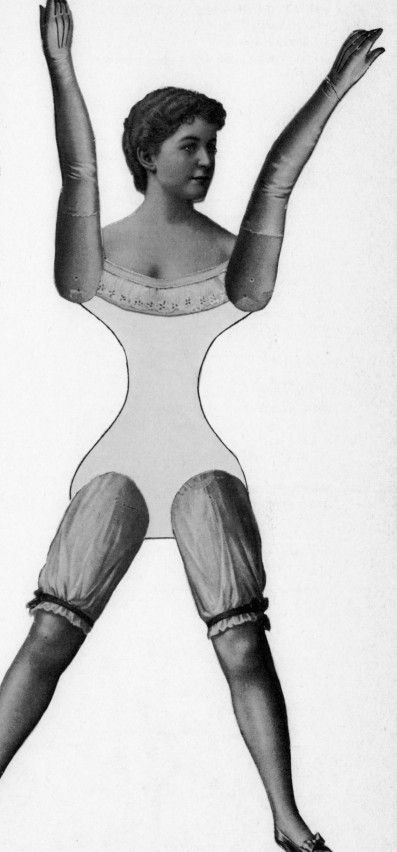

THE SENSUOUS APPROACH TO LOOKING YOUNGER
by Jessica Krane
$1.50 Paperback 149 pages Signet Books

Strictly speaking, this isn't a diet book, but it does have one chapter that speaks very directly about how we eat. Eating at the speed of a hurricane is one of the biggest problems I have—I get so excited when I see a plate of food that I almost pick up the whole plate and slide it into my mouth at one time. Jessica Krane's chapter on diet features a system called "Fletcherism" that swept the country many years ago.

According to Ms. Krane, in 1909 a man named Horace Fletcher was turned down for a life insurance policy when he was forty years old, because he was fifty pounds overweight. In desperation, he developed a new system of eating which is summed up in these lines,

Nature will castigate
Those who don't masticate.

In other words, we are to chew, chew, *chew* a certain number of times until the food becomes liquid and we extract all the flavor. To test this method, the War Department picked out thirty West Point cadets. They were taught Fletcherism and "as the weeks passed the researchers found the cadets drilling 'with a vigor and strength never before shown.' " The system seemed to be a success (obviously if you eat more slowly you'll eat less food); Fletcher lost sixty-five pounds, gained many honorary degrees, and became a celebrity.

CELLULITE
by Nicole Ronsard
$1.95 and $5.95 Paperback Bantam Books
(These books are exactly the same. One is pocket size, the other is much larger.)

This is the big cellulite book—sold 500,000 copies.

In 1967 Mme. Ronsard opened her now-famous Salon in New York City, the first in America devoted to the treatment of cellulite. She defines cellulite as: "gel-like lumps composed of fat, water, and the residues of toxic substances that should be—but have not been—eliminated by the body" and that lodge just below the surface of the skin—most likely in the thighs and buttocks. According to this book, there are six steps to eliminate this condition: proper diet, increasing the body's elimination, correct breathing, exercise geared to the trouble spots, massage, and relaxation. And it won't go away with an ordinary reducing diet and standard exercises.

I don't like to tell you this, but cellulite is primarily a feminine problem (though men may sometimes find it on the stomach and the nape of the neck). Why women? According to Ms. Ronsard, "In general, normal fat represents 24% of a woman's weight and only 11% of a man's." (Excuse me for a minute, I have to go look in the mirror.)

She also writes about the cellulite diet, "Purification and elimination are its primary goals, not weight loss."

In Ms. Ronsard's anti-cellulite diet, you are to eat plenty of fresh fruits and vegetables,

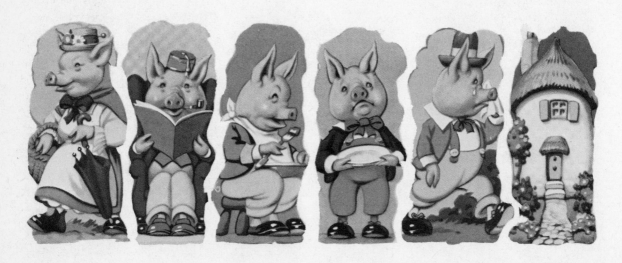

preferably at every meal. Have meat, poultry, and fish no more than once a day—preferably every other day. Don't use the salt-shaker too much, and drink six to eight glasses of water throughout the day.

HOW TO BE CELLULITE FREE FOREVER
by Susan Winer
$1.50 Paperback 218 pages Dell Books

Right on the first page of the book, Susan Winer brings up the earth-shattering question that has kept you up at night; does cellulite exist? She calls our attention to the controversy when she says she has "compiled very accurate and thorough research to enable you to draw your own conclusions about cellulite, its causes and its cures." I think that's very honest and upfront of Ms. Winer.

For this report, let us assume that cellulite does exist. Now that we agree on that, what *is* cellulite? According to the author, cellulite is fat, water, and wastes which stay in the connective tissues directly under the skin, causing the skin to have a soft, dimpled appearance—like the skin of an orange.

Okay, so we've got it. How do we get rid of it? Ms. Winer suggests a diet that is nutritionally balanced, with plenty of proteins, large amounts of water, and very little salt. Proteins help dissolve cellulite. They also stop water from collecting in the tissues. Water flushes the system of excess salt which could be trapped in the tissues. Salt causes a buildup of stagnant water in the body, which can be eliminated by using less salt.

There is no calorie-counting, unless you're on a calorie-counting diet already. Instead, you limit your food intake to meats, except pork and filled meats; poultry, except duck and goose; fish, except those that are smoked or cured, shellfish, and fish canned in oil; dairy products, except whole milk products, including ice cream, processed cheeses, and butter; various fruits and vegetables; whole-grained cereal products; water, tea, coffee, and sugar-free soda; you avoid liquor, beer, ale, and all sugar-sweetened soda pop.

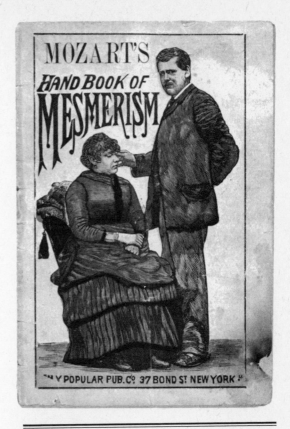

SELF HYPNOTISM
THE TECHNIQUE AND ITS USE IN DAILY LIVING
by Leslie M. LeCron, Clinical Psychologist
$1.50 Paperback 208 pages Signet Books

This is another book about why we overeat; the author feels we must know the reasons before we can lose weight and lose it permanently.

Some of the causes of overweight, he says, are lack of motivation, identity problems, and feelings of inferiority and unworthiness—all of them resulting in compulsive overeating. To overcome them the author gives you a step-by-step method of self-hypnosis, telling you how to induce self-hypnosis, how to measure the depth of hypnosis, and how to awaken yourself relaxed and refreshed, among other things. But *Self Hypnotism* is not primarily a diet book; it deals with all forms of compulsive behavior.

I must admit I've never tried self-hypnosis according to LeCron's methods. The closest I came was when I was eight years old and saw my first banana split. I was in a trance for a week.

INSPIRATION AND EXAMPLE

Any time I can find someone who has conquered a very difficult problem in their lives, I can't wait to talk to them or read how they did it. These folks have been through it. They're like a road map through uncharted, dangerous territory. Also they inspire, because they've been successful.

We all know how tough it is to lose weight and keep if off. To me there's nothing more inspiring than a former fatty who has taken all that dumb weight and cast it to the winds (so to speak).

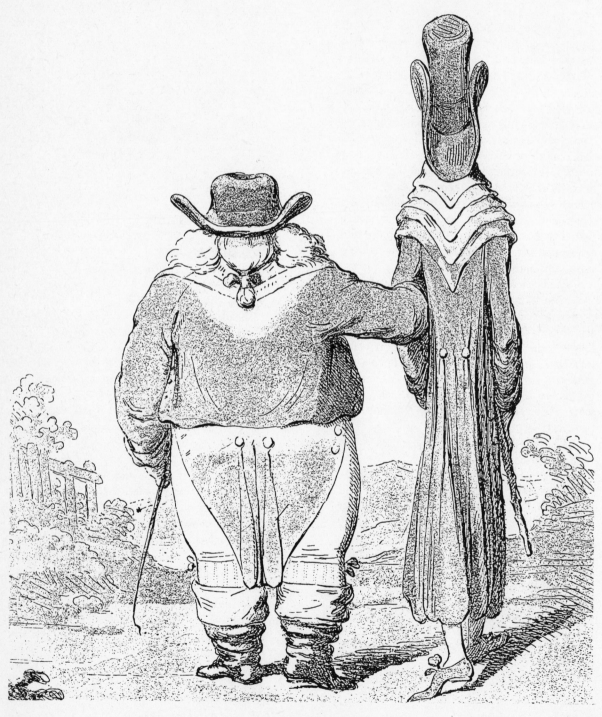

THE STORY OF WEIGHT WATCHERS
by Jean Nidetch as told to Joan Rattner Heilman
$1.25 Paperback 176 pages Signet Books

For all you Weight Watchers watchers, this is the story you've been waiting for: the journey of your beautiful slim guru from a fat 214-pound housewife to a 142-pound woman who founded Weight Watchers on principles she learned from her own dieting trials.

Jean Nidetch's story is fascinating even if, like me, you've never been or plan to be a Weight Watcher. It reads like the biography of most overweight people I know, including myself.

The "Fat Cell" of what was to become Weight Watchers started in 1961, when Ms. Nidetch got together with "six fat friends" to talk over their problems with losing weight and discuss her ten-week diet program from the New York City Department of Health's Obesity Clinic. (The Obesity Clinic is no longer in existence.)

The Story of Weight Watchers has "before" and "after" photos of Jean Nidetch and her family, a partial transcription of an actual class, and the Weight Watchers diet.

The book is very candid and honest, and in its own way, is a wonderful adventure story.

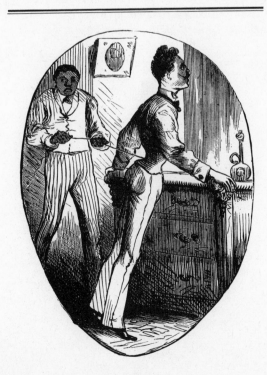

THEY LOST TWO TONS
SUCCESS STORIES FROM WEIGHT WATCHERS MAGAZINE
With a Foreword by Jean Nidetch
$1.50 Paperback 233 pages Warner Paperback Library

"How I Did It" stories always keep my eyes glued to the page and reading as fast as I can. It's inspiring to read about people who have struggled, fought, sweated, and finally succeeded at anything. This is doubly true about diet success stories. I always figure that someone else has discovered something about losing weight that heretofore was unknown.

In *They Lost Two Tons,* there are plenty of success stories we can empathize with. You can read how four nuns lost weight, about Charles Nelson Reilly, Ruth Buzzi, and Dom De Luise, and about a woman in Los Angeles who lost 312½ pounds. And besides the stories, there are incredible "before" and "after" pictures.

MEDICAL REPORTS FROM WEIGHT WATCHERS MAGAZINE
Foreword by Jean Nidetch
$1.50 Paperback 205 pages Signet Books

This book is a compilation of medical reports that originally appeared in *Weight Watchers Magazine.*

I always thought *Dracula* and *Psycho* were the scariest things I'd ever seen in my life. That was until I picked up this little number. After reading just the table of contents, they made those two horror films look like *Boys' Life* and *Heidi.*

Strap yourself in your chair and I'll give you a few samples of the articles: Obesity and Emotional Illness, Obesity and the Unborn Child, Diabetes Pursues Obesity, Obesity and Heart Trouble, and Obesity and Varicose Veins.

This is strong medicine—if it doesn't convince you to watch your weight, it could just scare the fat right off.

ASK JEAN
QUESTIONS TO JEAN NIDETCH, FOUNDER OF WEIGHT WATCHERS INTERNATIONAL
$1.75 Paperback 169 pages Signet Books

1. **"Dear Jean:** I know you travel a lot and speak to many people. I am curious to know what question is asked of you most often?"
2. **"Dear Jean:** I see many ads for certain pills and reducing machines and other products that guarantee weight loss. Does the Weight Watchers Program guarantee loss?"
3. **"Dear Jean:** My lecturer tells me I must eat fish 5 times a week. I don't like fish. I never eat fish. Isn't there some other food I can possibly substitute?"*

These are some of the hundreds of questions asked Jean Nidetch. (If you want to know the answers, see below.)

I've always been a sucker for questions and answers about anything, but especially about dieting. Maybe I like them because I ask a million questions in everyday life. Here the questions you want to ask about weight loss are broken down into categories: General, Program, Food, Problems, Humor or a Lighter Approach, and Love Letters.

This book has a lot of good information, plus amazing "before" and "after" pictures of some of the successful W.W. members.

WEIGHT WATCHERS MAGAZINE
635 Madison Avenue
New York, New York 10022
Phone: (212) 838-8964
75¢ at your newsdealer or by subscription

Weight Watchers Magazine is in a class by it-self—quite literally, because it's the only one in its class. Although there are annual diet magazines, this is the only monthly magazine I've been able to find that specializes in weight reduction.

There are articles on fashion, belly dancing, what to do about wrinkling, how Shirley MacLaine got to be trim and terrific, what makes good food taste good, plus many, many recipes, as well as the latest news from the diet world. There are regular features such as "Ask Joan"—answers to readers' questions about dieting; "Girtha," a comic strip about an overweight woman; and a reader-recipe of the month. In the ten or twelve issues I've read, success stories about people who have lost weight and kept it off are an important part of each issue. They, like the before and after pictures also provided, are an inspiration to the overweight reader.

In my opinion, the magazine is aimed primarily at women. As for us fat (and formerly fat but still weight-obsessed) guys—there doesn't seem to be anything directed to us. Until there is, *Weight Watchers Magazine* provides an enormous boost for overweight folks, male and female, who need all the help they can get.

---

*ANSWERS

1. "What do you when you get a craving for fattening foods?" Jean's reply: "I take a bubble bath. I do something that I really enjoy."
2. "As far as I'm concerned, no one but you could guarantee weight loss. We guarantee nothing except that you will have a food plan that is well balanced and that you can stick with, and that you will meet and talk to other people who have the same needs as yours."
3. "Fish is one of the most nutritious, high-protein foods available. It is a great aid in weight loss and can be quite satisfying. Eat fish."

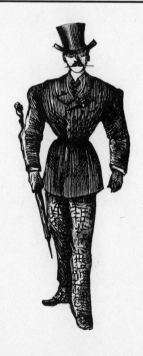

COSMOPOLITAN'S SUPER DIETS & EXERCISE GUIDE
$1.50 Magazine 96 pages

Cosmo has really wrapped it up for you in only ninety-six pages. Just look what you get: thirteen diets guaranteed to work, eleven ways to exercise your body, five ways to exercise your mind (and lose weight), seven ways to keep your health while dieting, lots of questions and answers about dieting, seventy-five diet menus and recipes, and, to top it off, a complete calorie-counter.

Cosmopolitan magazine has done a tremendous job. *Super Diets and Exercise Guide* has taken the whole weight-reducing and exercise field, digested it, and given you the newest and best.

Besides all the helpful words, guys, there's a lot of appealing pictures of those beautiful *Cosmo* women. I especially liked the shot of a woman in a kitchen mixing up a cake. I certainly would like to help *her* sift the flour.

Of course, the diet I liked best is "The Aphrodisiac Diet for Lovers." Don't giggle. *Cosmopolitan* got none other than Fredrick J. Stare, M.D., Professor of Nutrition and Chairman of Harvard University's Department of Nutrition, to design the diet.

Among the many foods that Dr. Stare says have supposedly aphrodisiac properties are oysters, caviar, and asparagus. Now, I'm expecting a little somebody in a few minutes and I have 43 pounds of asparagus boiling on the stove.

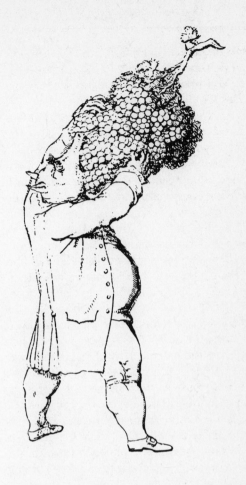

GOD'S ANSWER TO FAT, LOSE IT!
by Frances Hunter
Foreword by Graham Kerr
$2.95 Paperback 147 pages Hunter Ministries

The titles of this book's thirteen chapters tell you what the book is about: "The Great Christian Fib," "The Great Awakening," "How Did It Start And Where Does It End?," "Wisdom And Knowledge Come Galloping In," "Gluttony," "Where Do We Go From Here?," "The Devil Is A 'Sweet' Liar," "The Great Substitution," "Learn the Law!," "Why Don't I 'Want' To Lose Weight?," "The Wrap Up," "Nutritive Value of Foods," and "Skinny Minnie Recipes."

Frances Hunter had tried almost every kind of diet and exercise regimen with no permanent success. She always gained all the weight she lost right back. But, as she says on the book jacket, "Your appetite can be healed! Discover that God wants to take away that 'fat' appetite and give you a slender one!"

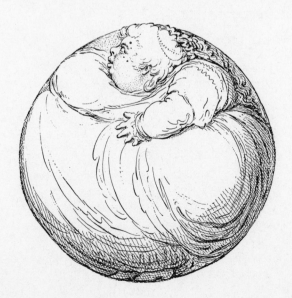

THE BEAUTIFUL PEOPLE'S DIET BOOK
by Luciana Avedon and Jeanne Molli
$1.50 Paperback 146 pages Bantam Books

The Beautiful People's Diet Book is a juicy weight reducer. It's loaded with gossip about the Beautiful People and how they diet—whoever the Beautiful People are. I'm sorry to say I don't personally know the Hon. Mrs. Vere (Pat) Harmsworth, Baroness Gaby Van Zuylen, or Giorgio Sant'Angelo, but I must be hanging out at the wrong joints.

The authors say they talked to the Beautiful People because they have their weight visibly under control and they can't afford to be fat. (They don't say anything about all of us Ugly People.) Of the people they interviewed, the society columnist, Suzy, says when she's five pounds over she cuts back to 1000 calories a day. Betsy Bloomingdale says when she's two pounds over she eats half of everything until she's back to normal. Françoise de la Renta lives on three quarts of vegetable bouillon one day a week. And Merle Oberon lives on yogurt, raisins, and almonds for a day or two, along with vitamins and additional protein powder in the yogurt.

The book also tells you what fat farms the B.P. go to, what they feed their children, what they think about "natural" foods and their diets, and what's going on in Europe in the weight-reducing world.

What it all boils down to is that in order to get slim and trim the Beautiful People have to eat less food and get more exercise, just as we do. But somehow it sounds like more fun when they do it.

DEVOTIONS FOR DIETERS
by Reverend H. Victor Kane
95¢ Paperback 64 pages Spire Books

Devotions for Dieters was written by Reverend H. Victor Kane, himself a successful dieter. The book contains six weeks of reading material, divided week by week into devotions, suggestions, parables, graces, and poetry.

Let me give you one of the table graces for dieters:

"O God, accept my thanks for health,
Above all else, the truest wealth;
Help me to guard it day by day
By eating in a prudent way. Amen."

As Reverend Kane says, "The real motivation for losing weight and keeping it off must come from within each dieter." Amen.

Who holds the record for eating? According to medical texts, Matthew Daking, age 12, in 1743 consumed 384 pounds of food in six days.

DIET COOKBOOKS

Cookbooks in general are fascinating reading. Especially if you enjoy food vicariously. Diet cookbooks in particular offer one of the most creative sections of the weight-reducing world. I'm always amazed at the variety and number of delicious-sounding low-calorie recipes that most of them contain. Many of these books have grown out of the programs of diet groups, or out of other successful diet books.

As for myself, I literally do not have a pot or a pan. Sounds funny for a food man like me, but I'm not thrilled with cooking. After slaving over a hot pizza oven all day, I've had enough. Judging from the wealth of cookbooks available, however, I'm in the great minority. Most men and women get a charge out of imaginative cooking and serving, and with these cookbooks they can feed themselves or their families delicious low-calorie meals.

By the way, if you have an extra chair at your dining table, I'm always available.

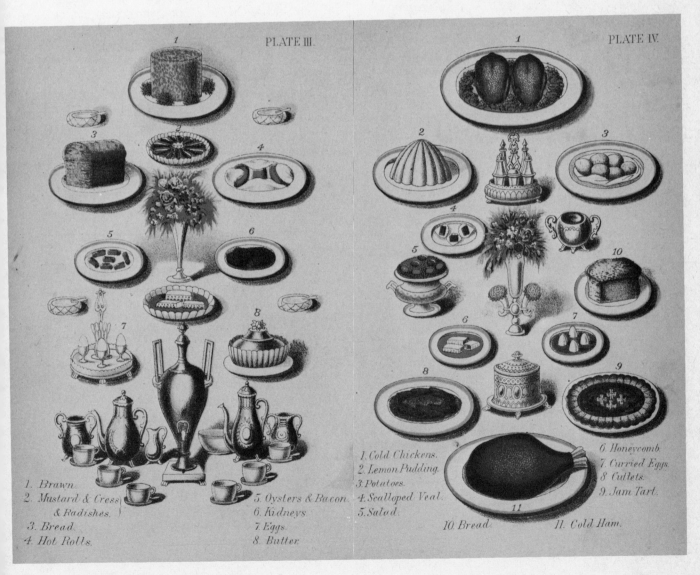

PLATE III.

1. Brawn.
2. Mustard & Cress & Radishes.
3. Bread.
4. Hot Rolls.
5. Oysters & Bacon.
6. Kidneys.
7. Eggs.
8. Butter.

PLATE IV.

1. Cold Chickens.
2. Lemon Pudding.
3. Potatoes.
4. Scalloped Veal.
5. Salad.
6. Honeycomb.
7. Curried Eggs.
8. Cutlets.
9. Jam Tart.
10. Bread.
11. Cold Ham.

BETTER HOMES AND GARDENS CALORIE COUNTER'S COOK BOOK
$1.25 Paperback 164 pages Bantam Books

The Better Homes and Gardens Calorie Counter's Cook Book has been through seven printings since 1972 and is the recipient of a big plug from the Council of Foods and Nutrition of the American Medical Association. All the recipes therein have been "tested for family appeal, practicality and deliciousness, and endorsed by the Better Homes and Gardens Test Kitchen."

There are "Calorie-Trimmed Recipes" for appetizers and snacks, main dishes, vegetables, salads, sandwiches, desserts, beverages; low-calorie menus; and sections on low-calorie entertaining and how to maintain your weight with helpful hints and a calorie chart.

The recipes have such glorious names as Fruited Chicken Breasts (157 calories a serving); Shrimp-Mushroom Soufflé (202 calories a serving); Sunshine Apple Mold (80 calories a serving); and my favorite, Mocha Chiffon, "a rich, flavorful blend of cocoa and coffee" (104 calories a serving).

DR. ATKINS' DIET COOKBOOK
by Fran Gare and Helen Monica, under the supervision of and with an introduction by Robert C. Atkins, M.D.
$1.95 Paperback 291 pages Bantam Books

All you experienced dieters who've ever breezed through the diet-book section of your local book emporium know about Dr. Atkins and his Diet Revolution (see page 12). And if you've never bought a diet book in your life, you must have friends who have been on the "Atkins Diet." As the doctor himself describes it: "On this diet you don't watch calories, you watch carbohydrates."

Dr. Atkins' Diet Cookbook has a twenty-one-day recipe program offering you luxurious delicacies like Crabmeat Almond Pie, Baked Ham Soufflé, Pizza with Meat Crust, Fresh Spring Salmon Mousse, Cannelloni with Chicken, and Strawberry-Lemon Meringue Pie. Look at some of the ingredients the various recipes call for: heavy cream, butter, Parmesan cheese, crisp bacon, more heavy cream, lobster meat, olive oil, fried pork rinds, sour cream, egg yolks, and *more* heavy cream. Now that's fancy eatin'.

There are over 300 recipes, plus a restaurant menus guide to eating dietetically in ethnic—and other—restaurants. Chinese, French, Italian, Greek, Spanish, as well as vegetarian and dairy and, my favorite kind of ethnic eating, Steak House—are all included.

THE DOCTOR'S QUICK WEIGHT LOSS DIET COOKBOOK
by Irwin Maxwell Stillman, M.D., and Samm Sinclair Baker
$1.75 Paperback 346 pages Bantam Books

The Doctor's Quick Weight Loss Diet Cookbook includes 600 recipes for the famous Quick Weight Loss, Teen Quick Weight Loss, and Inches-Off Diets, along with descriptions of the three diets, so you can check what you're cooking. (Obviously you should see your doctor before starting anything.)

The recipes run the whole gamut from hors d'oeuvres and dips through desserts and beverages, with low-calorie versions of Veal Scallopine with Wine Sauce, Cold Shellfish Salad, Poached Pears, and Home-Style Pineapple Sherbet. Also included are plan-ahead menus, money- and calorie-saving tips, ideal-weight and calorie charts, and a guide list of herbs and spices.

THE SLIM GOURMET COOKBOOK
by Barbara Gibbons
$12.95 Hardbound 401 pages Harper & Row

Barbara Gibbons, herself an ex-heavyweight and now the author of the nationally syndicated column "Slim Gourmet," once tipped the scales at 208. Here she gives tips that she discovered and tested in her kitchen: by "de-calorizing" fattening favorites, she eliminated hundreds of calories a day that nobody will ever miss, and created a wonderful diet cookbook. In each recipe she shows how to use ingredients that taste the same as their more fattening friends, yet have fewer calories, and the results are chili con carne with only 250 calories a serving, crab Newburg (150 calories), chopped chicken livers (only 80 calories), and cheesecake made with farmer cheese (136 calories). There is a five-day menu plan that includes dishes like "Cordon Bleu" veal (271 calories), spaghetti and meatballs (350 calories), and a chocolate milkshake (90 calories).

This book begins with low-calorie appetizers such as cheese-stuffed mushrooms (15 calories) and goes on to cover every course, including spaghetti dishes, jellies, breads, cakes, pies, and beverages.

More than a cookbook, it's a how-to manual for calorie-coping in the supermarket, equipping your kitchen, and eating out in restaurants and at dinner parties without gaining weight.

DIET FOR ONE, DINNER FOR ALL
by Beryl M. Marton
$7.95 Hardbound 165 pages Golden Press

"Good Evening and welcome to Beryl Marton's *Diet for One, Dinner for All.* I am your waiter, Laurent Goldberg.

"The choices tonight are Shrimp Remoulade, Asparagus Parmesan, Coq au Vin, Veal Ragout, Bananas Flambés, and Rum Sauce.

"Here you will find no fad diets, no dietetic products and no sugar substitutes in any of the foods or menus. And each gourmet menu is around 500 calories.

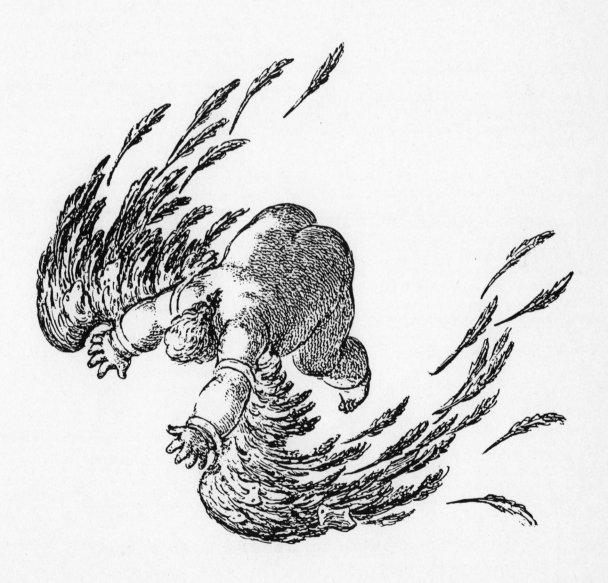

"If tonight's menu doesn't please you, let me whet your appetite with tomorrow's 531-calorie dinner.

Crabmeat-Stuffed Cherry Tomatoes
Duck à l'Orange
Wild Rice
Green Beans Lyonnaise
Dessert Fondue

"Yes, of course, you may bring in your nondieting husband, children, friends, lovers, relatives or clergyman. That is the purpose of *Diet for One, Dinner for All*. Whether you're on a diet or not, anyone can enjoy all those scrumptious menus.

"And *Diet for One, Dinner for All* won the 1974 R.T. French Tastemaker Award in the Health and Diet Category and is a Literary Cook Book Guild Selection.

"Your table is waiting."

FOOD & COOKING FOR HEALTH
by Lawrence E. Lamb, M.D.
$4.95 Hardbound 412 pages A Viking Compass Book

A one-and-a-half-inch thick, near-encyclopedia of food information which features caloric and nutritional analyses as well as 300 recipes. The first half of the book involves what amounts to a bachelor's degree in food and nutrition; then there is information on how to plan a diet, followed by recipes.

Food and Cooking for Health is organized as a progression of steps. As the author says, "Each chapter builds on the information that has preceded it. To illustrate: when you reach the salad chapter, you will already have covered the chapters on vegetables, fruits and salad dressings." The recipes themselves don't conform to any particular diet ideology—Dr. Lamb says, "You can follow a low-calorie diet, a low-fat diet, a low-saturated fat diet, a balanced ratio of polyunsaturated fat to saturated fat, a low-cholesterol diet, or any combination of these."

THE NEW YORK TIMES NATURAL FOODS DIETING BOOK
by Yvonne Young Tarr
$1.95 Paperback 303 pages Ballantine Books

The title of the book tells us all. Ms. Tarr says that we must eat natural foods high in vitamins and minerals and give up those nasty additives, preservatives, artificial colorings, and chemicals. If we do this, our unnatural cravings for sweets and starches will disappear, and "losing weight becomes easier and pleasanter than you ever thought possible." This is the way Ms. Tarr dieted, so she ought to know.

The first twenty-four pages deal with various "natural" diets, including the Substitution Method, the Low Calorie Method, the Low Calorie Diet, Low Calorie Maintenance, the Low Carbohydrate Diet, and Low Carbohydrate Maintenance.

The rest of the book is recipes, ranging from Homemade Cottage Cheese (1 pint sour milk plus sea salt to taste) to Brain Salad (don't ask). In between are dishes like Skewered Chicken Livers, Apples with Honey, Dill Butter, Banana Cole Slaw, and Strawberry Yogurt Sherbet. Each and every recipe has the calories and carbohydrates listed, and there are also nutrition charts.

Additional information is included on where to find natural foods, and on buying natural and organic foods by mail.

If you want to get into natural foods and you're a little on the chunky side, this is an appealing, well-researched book—but keep your eye on the recipes. They look delicious, but some are loaded with calories.

"The fat man knoweth not what the lean thinketh."
—George Herbert

HELEN CORBITT COOKS FOR LOOKS
by Helen Corbitt
$5.95 Hardbound 115 pages Houghton Mifflin

Helen Corbitt is the director of restaurants at Neiman-Marcus in Dallas, Texas. She was also asked to plan the meals for The Greenhouse, an elegant beauty spa for women in Arlington, Texas, and now she has produced a cookbook beautiful both outside and inside. The cover is a pale lime green that is very soothing to the feverish dieter's brow.

Ms. Corbitt doesn't believe in loading up at breakfast. A little fresh fruit, black coffee or tea, one slice of melba toast that you make yourself, and, if that isn't enough, a poached or boiled egg ("leave the yolk in the dish")—that's all. Therefore, all the menus and recipes (four weeks' worth) deal with lunch and dinner and special events. Each day's menu is planned to have only 850 calories, which can include such delicacies as Cold Lemon Soufflé, Artichokes Stuffed with Shrimp and Hearts of Palm, and Roast Capon with Truffle Sauce. All of the recipes have been tried out at The Greenhouse, where the average weight loss is five to seven pounds per week.

With this book, you can have your very own luxury spa in your house. The diet menus are in the book, exercises can be done on the new living-room carpeting, and your spouse or a close friend can give you the massage. See, this book has already saved you a few thousand bucks.

100 DELICIOUS WAYS TO STAY SLIM
by Shirley Bright Boody
75¢ Paperback 203 pages Award Books

A handy little book that contains 100 complete menus for breakfasts, lunches, suppers, dinner parties, and what to feed teenagers. There's practical advice on how to make mealtimes more enjoyable, what to eat between meals, and how much to eat to control weight.

Each menu plan contains the recipes to prepare a meal like the following: Iced Crab Cocktail, Chicken Breasts Florentine, Creamed Artichoke Hearts, Carmel Baked Tomatoes, Maple Mousse, and beverage. Ms. Boody uses ordinary foods, emphasizing good seasoning and preparation and careful meal-planning. She shows you ways to put nonfattening zip into old favorites and new pizzazz into meal-times. Her cry is, "Cook Skinny." Right on.

THE BRAND-NAME DIET
by Jean Sommers
$1.25 Paperback 190 pages Award Books

This is for the dieter who wants both convenience and low calories: a collection of recipes that use brand-name supermarket foods—canned, frozen, ready-to-serve packaged products—in various low-calorie recipes.

You can choose brand-name products from such companies as Campbell's, Durkee, Birds Eye, Dole, Chun King, and Banquet.

I'll give you the ingredients for Old-Fashioned Meat Loaf to show you how it works: one can Campbell's Condensed Vegetable Soup; two and a half pounds lean ground beef; one cup chopped onion; three-quarters cup dry bread crumbs; one egg, slightly beaten; one teaspoon salt; dash of pepper—makes eight servings at 231 calories each. You can also make such gourmet goodies as Caviar Eggs Tartare, Broiled Cranburgers, Dieter's Blue Cheese Dressing, and Holiday Apple Pie (170 calories a slice).

There are also daily menu plans of 1200, 1500, 1800, or 2100 calories, using the recipes in the book.

This is a terrific idea for a diet cookbook. It's easy, low-calorie, and much of the work is done for you. Now if Ms. Sommers could just get rid of those long lines in the supermarkets . . .

Diet Watchers groups use a diet similar to the diet published by the New York City Health Department. Diet Watchers is discussed in greater detail elsewhere in this catalog (see page 70). Anyway, the two Diet Watchers cookbooks can be used by anyone trying to lose weight.

THE DIET WATCHERS GOURMET COOKBOOK
by Ann Gold and Sarah Welles Briller
$1.95 Paperback 160 pages Grosset & Dunlap

All you folks who love international cooking but have to keep an eye on the scale should have a good time with this one. There are recipes for breakfasts, lunches, dinners, main dishes, vegetables, side dishes, salads, and sauces. And, slim globe-trotter, these include recipes from Italian, French, Jewish, Scandinavian, Russian, Middle Eastern, Oriental, Canadian, Latin, and American cuisines. Pack your bags and fly into the kitchen.

THE DIET WATCHERS DESSERT COOKBOOK
by Ann Gold
$1.95 Paperback 120 pages Grosset & Dunlap

Sweet tooth as big as the Grand Canyon? This book can give you a jolt like hot fudge at a fraction of the calories, with 160 super recipes for beverages, breads, candies, cakes, cookies, fruit desserts, ice cream, ices, and sherbets, parfaits, mousses and molded desserts, puddings and pies, tarts and turnovers, jams, preserves, sauces, and snacks.

THE EPICURE'S VERY LOW CARBOHYDRATE COOKBOOK
by Marilyn Van Syckel
$2.50 Paperback 244 pages Barnes and Noble

This is a cookbook for the thousands of people who have lost weight on the Atkins, Stillman, or "Drinking Man's" low-carbohydrate diets, and want to keep it off.

There are recipes for everything from appetizers through desserts and the carbohydrate gram count is given with each recipe. Four hundred recipes are included, many from the finest restaurants in New York and San Francisco: You can dine on such gourmet dishes as Stuffed Mushrooms Parmigiana, Roast Pheasant with Madeira, and Strawberries Romanoff.

The great innovation in this book—the thing that sets it apart from other low-carbohydrate cookbooks—is that it contains a bread recipe that is low in carbohydrates. It uses cream of tartar as a leavening agent and soya powder, a high-protein nutrient, instead of flour.

LOW CARBOHYDRATE COOKBOOK
by Joanne Waring Lindeman
$3.95 Paperback 183 pages Nitty Gritty Productions

For you carbohydrate-counters, this is an ideal cookbook to give or receive. The recipes sound delicious, the type is big, the directions are simple, and the pages lie flat without your having to put a shot put on the crease.

There are recipes for everything: salads, sauces, dressings, meat, poultry, seafood, eggs, cheese, vegetables, and desserts. How about ham-stuffed mushrooms—1.1 grams of carbohydrate per serving—or filets with bernaise cream sauce or wild duck or chocolate torte at 2.7 grams per serving?

All these recipes for folks on low-carbohydrate diets drive me crazy. Every one sounds so fattening and yummy. But if you watch the carbos, you can eat all these goodies and still lose weight.

Sounds good to me.

THE LOW-CARBOHYDRATE DIETER'S COOKBOOK
by William Thorne
$1.25 Paperback 182 pages Pinnacle Books

William Thorne, a restaurateur, chef, and caterer, has developed 200 recipes based on Dr. Atkins' low-carbohydrate weight-reduction system. Mr. Thorne weighed 432 pounds and was 5'11" tall when he began the Atkins diet. "Within three months I had lost 93 pounds," he tells us. The book was copyrighted in 1973; let's hope Bill Thorne has continued his dramatic weight losses in the intervening years.

LOW CHOLESTEROL, LOWER CALORIE FRENCH COOKING
by Stanley Leinwoll
$6.95 Hardbound 147 pages Charles Scribners

For this book Stanley Leinwoll created recipes in which he makes substitutions for the cheese, butter, eggs, and cream that are a trademark of French cuisine. This reduces cholesterol to a minimum and lowers the calories without, he maintains, significantly changing the flavor of traditional French dishes. As a result, all the recipes "conform with standards of good eating practices as set forth by the American Heart Association."

There are gorgeous recipes for soups, sauces, fish and seafood, poultry, meat, vegetables, bread, and desserts. At the end of each recipe there are four listings: calories per serving, cholesterol count, saturated fats, and polyunsaturates.

All the dishes have long French names with English subtitles and each one made my mouth water although I'm the type who'd choose a cold sausage and onion pizza over a plateful of *coq au vin* any day. A well-researched, tempting collection of recipes.

THE CARBO-CALORIE DIET COOKBOOK
by Donald S. Mart
$1.95 Paperback 185 pages Dolphin Books

This cookbook includes 250 recipes for international and ethnic gourmet meals based on the Carbo-Calorie Diet. According to the author you must compute your calories / carbohydrates ratio (Carbo-Calories) with a mathematical formula. I'd like to tell you how to use the formula, but my experience with numbers is limited to adding up restaurant checks—and I still make mistakes. Anyway, you're supposed to keep your Carbo-Calories to a hundred or fewer per day, and these recipes can help you do that.

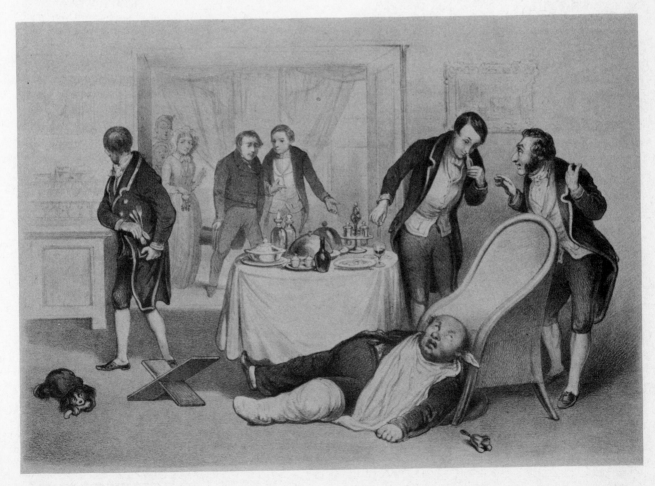

THE HIP, HIGH-PROTE, LOW-CAL, EASY-DOES-IT COOKBOOK
by Naura Hayden
$5.95 Hardbound 195 pages Dodd, Mead

"Don't Count Calories, Count Proteins"—that's what Naura Hayden tells us to do. According to her, we need a minimum of seventy grams of complete protein every day. But, she says, many people get only twenty-five grams. "No wonder muscles are saggy, colds are frequent, teeth are cavitied, skin is wrinkly, and nerves are bad." (I'm beginning to feel not so good just writing this.)

The Hip, High-Prote, Low-Cal, Easy-Does-It Cookbook has nearly 200 recipes that use no meat or sugar. Many recipes have eggs in them, so I guess it is not a strict vegetarian cookbook.

Chapter headings include "Dynamite for Breakfast," "Egg-O-Mania," "Snappy-Tizers," and "There's a Tiger in My Thoup" (soup, get it?). Each recipe includes its total calories and grams of complete protein.

I'll give you some highlights of the recipe called "Breakfast Cake Go-Go": half a cup soy powder, half a cup soy grits, half a cup noninstant powdered skim milk, half a cup wheat germ (untoasted), half a cup whole wheat flour, one cup sunflower seeds, half a cup sesame seeds, two and two-thirds teaspoons granulated sugar substitute, half a teaspoon sea salt, three eggs, half a cup skim milk, two tablespoons safflower oil, two tablespoons honey, and one cup fresh fruit (berries, apples, apricots, pears, peaches, etc.). Makes ten slices. Each slice has 17 grams of complete protein, 329 calories.

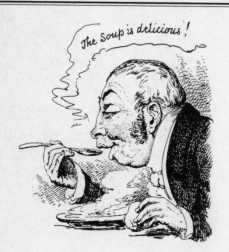

The soup is delicious!

THE WINE DIET COOKBOOK
by Dr. Salvatore P. Lucia and Emily Chase, M.S.
$8.95 Hardbound 132 pages Abelard-Schuman, Ltd.

For all you overweight winos, this diet could be the answer. Even if you're not a wino, this diet is a very elegant way to lose weight. As the authors point out, a glass of dry wine has about ninety calories, and they have included a glass of wine for dinner in all the menu plans in the book. The reason for this is that studies have shown that if you drink wine with your dinner you won't eat as much—besides, the wine has a tranquilizing effect, which will keep you from running amok in the refrigerator late at night. Wine also makes you sleep better—all of which is detailed in a fascinating section on how alcohol functions in your body.

Many of the recipes in the book call for wine as an ingredient, and the authors tell you not to worry about the sugar in wine when you're cooking, since wine will lose 85 percent of its sugar when cooked in sufficient heat. Wine, they conclude, is a good source of energy and contains usable vitamins and minerals, so you should think about including it in all sorts of diets.

The diet outlined in this book is a variation on our old friend the Prudent or New York City Health Department Diet. It allows you 1200 calories a day, including a four-ounce glass of table wine. The authors say that with a 1200-calorie diet, you are including all the elements for basic nutrition and you can average a two-pound weight loss a week.

The Wine Diet Cookbook gives you twenty-eight days of 1200-calorie menus and recipes for every dish. The recipes sound delicious—Braised Stuffed Flank Steak (257 calories per serving); Barbecued Chicken El Dorado (375 calories per serving); and, for dessert, Ambrosia (127 calories per serving). Here's the recipe for Ambrosia:

For each serving allow half a cup of fresh orange segments, one-quarter teaspoon grated orange peel, one tablespoon California muscatel, one-third cup ripe banana slices, and one teaspoon shredded coconut. Combine orange segments, orange peel, and wine; cover; chill. Just before serving, add banana slices; mix lightly; top with coconut. Garnish, if desired, with a no-calorie sprig of fresh mint. Only 127 calories.

THE SAVE-YOUR-LIFE-DIET HIGH-FIBER COOKBOOK
by David Reuben, M.D., and Barbara Reuben, M.S.
$7.95 Hardbound 213 pages Random House

According to the authors, "The menus and recipes and the philosophy of The Save-Your-Life High-Fiber Cookbook are designed to enable everyone to reproduce the diet that Americans consumed a hundred years ago—before 750,000 of us perished each year from heart attacks, before one of us succumbed to colon cancer every ten minutes by the clock, before seventy percent of those who collect Social Security also collect diverticulosis, before over half of us had our bodies bloated by ugly fat."

Boy, Dr. Reuben ought to be writing for Alfred Hitchcock. He scared me enough in his first book, *The Save-Your-Life Diet* (see page 14): I started eating bran over a year ago and am still going strong. Now, in a natural follow-up to that hugely successful first book, he tells you how to make all sorts of high-fiber dishes. The recipes are easy to follow and include grains, bread and pastries, meat, poultry and fish, vegetables, eggs and cheese, pasta, soups, salads, desserts, and even candy (but keep a sharp eye on the ingredients to make sure they're nonfattening).

As the Reubens point out, bran can be included in nearly every weight-reduction program. You can read the first book to find Dr. Reuben's high-roughage reducing diet. It is briefly discussed in this book too.

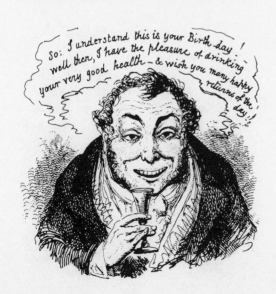

So: I understand this is your Birth day! Well then, I have the pleasure of drinking your very good health - & wish you many happy returns of the day!

CUISINE MINCEUR—THE CUISINE OF SLIMNESS
by Michel Guerard
$12.95 Hardbound 320 pages Morrow

This is the big one—the gourmet diet cookbook by the chef who has "revolutionized" French cooking and garnered praise from every gourmet writer from here to your Cuisinart.

Anyway, Michel Guerard's *Cuisine Minceur* (pronounced *man-sir*) is a new concept in French cooking, a method of preparing French food with far fewer calories by staying away from fats and carbohydrates and concentrating on the "essences" of meats, fish, fresh vegetables, and fruits. Guerard's menus are planned to put you on a 1000-calorie-a-day diet, and the only special equipment you need is sharp knives, a blender, and a Teflon pan. Every lunch and dinner is a three-course meal, ending with a dessert made with an artificial sweetener.

You may dine on fish steamed on a bed of herbs, poached chicken in terrines with crayfish, oranges with candied rinds, and a pear soufflé that puffs up in the oven but not on your hips. And there are many more low-calorie dishes and menus.

THE EAT-TO-LOSE COOKBOOK
by Ceil Dyer
$7.95 Hardbound 151 pages Mason/Charter

You can cook up a four-wind storm with this book. For sumptuous dining without adding the poundage, choose from French, Italian, Oriental, and Californian (whatever that is) cuisines.

Just think—you can have café au lait for breakfast, a lunch of Italian antipasto, and stir-fry chicken with almonds for dinner.

All the recipes are low-calorie and based on sound principles of good nutrition. So you can eat well, get all the necessary vitamins and minerals, and still lose weight.

According to the author, this is a diet recipe program to help you lose weight and keep it off the rest of your life.

HOW TO USE SUGAR TO LOSE WEIGHT
by June Roth
95¢ Paperback 157 pages Award Books

You say you like sugar? You say you're tired of those bland old diet foods? You say you need a little sugar fix every once in a while? Grab this book.

According to the author, "The purpose of this book is to give you a variety of recipes using small amounts of natural sugar in all forms."

She also says, "It is foolish to make sugar the culprit for overeating and bad food choices." Now that's fair. She also points out that sugar has only eighteen calories a teaspoon, and is also an effective energy-producer and taste-improver.

Ms. Roth has developed recipes for Trim Tempters, Skinny Soups, Melting Mainstays, Vain Vegetables, and Deft Desserts. You can dine on such sweet goodnesses as Chicken Luau, sweetened with pineapple chunks, brown sugar, and ground ginger (235 calories per serving) or Lemon Sponge Cake, sweetened with a cup of sugar (113 calories per serving).

This is a fascinating diet concept and if, like me, you're hooked on sugar, this could be a great deal of help. But be careful and selective in the recipes you use, you sweet thing, you.

THE COMPLETE YOGURT COOKBOOK
by Karen Cross Whyte
$1.50 Paperback 160 pages Ballantine Books

Open this book with caution. There's a lot of yummy high-calorie recipes for all sorts of yogurt dishes in here. But you're smart enough to know the fattening ones from the skinnies.

I included this book because there are many delicious low-calorie recipes for such dishes as Frosty Cucumber Soup, Tangy Braised Beef Cubes, and Slim Shortcake, as well as information on the history of yogurt, yogurt folklore, how yogurt is made commercially, and how to make yogurt at home.

Many of the people I know who are always on diets think yogurt is a magic elixir that can help cure everything from athlete's foot to whisker burn. Whatever it does for you, it sure is popular, tangy, and refreshing and takes a long time to eat. But be careful what you add to the plain yogurt or you might as well eat a chocolate ice cream soda.

MAKING YOUR OWN BABY FOOD
by Mary Turner and James Turner
$1.25 Paperback 128 pages Bantam Books

My mother told me that when I was a baby, I was eating so much she couldn't give me enough milk, so she stopped breast-feeding me and started me on cereals at an incredibly

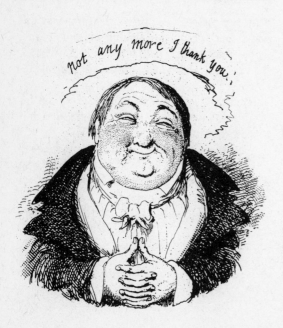

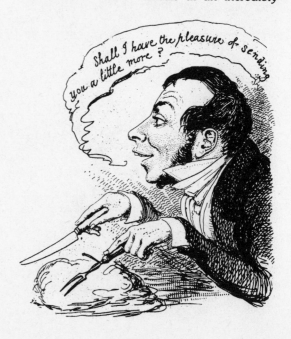

young age. According to some experts, that's when my fat problems could have started; but now you can start your children off on the right foot with a nutritional, nonfattening diet with food you make yourself.

The two authors of this book are a husband-and-wife team: James Turner is the author of the 1970 Nader report on the Food and Drug Administration, *The Chemical Feast;* Mary Turner began to devise her own recipes for baby food when her husband was away on a sea tour and she and her six-month-old son moved in with her mother, aunt, and grandmother, who "weren't having any part of modern baby feeding methods." By talking with them, reading about natural foods, and experimenting, Ms. Turner developed her own program of feeding.

Making Your Own Baby Food includes the latest thinking on feeding babies properly, and tells you where to buy and how to make wholesome baby foods without going broke. In addition, because a baby's health is so dependent on its mother's health, there is a section on prenatal health. There are also recipes for fruits, vegetables, meats, and snacks.

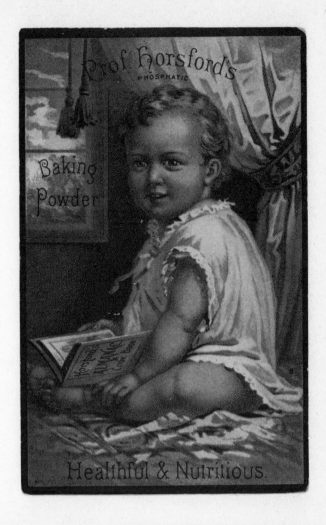

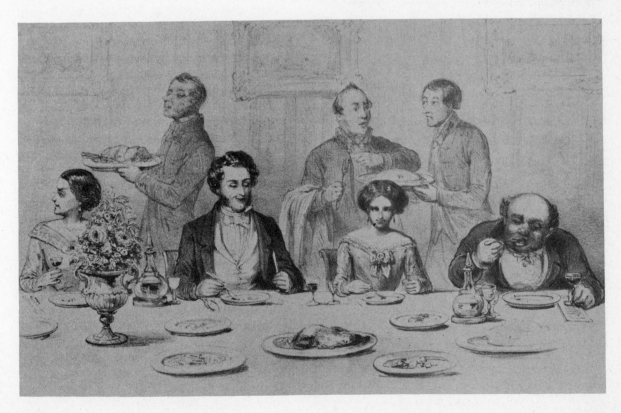

THE CHEF'S DESSERT COOKBOOK
by Dominque D'Ermo
$12.50 Hardbound 350 pages
   Atheneum

Don't look at the photo of the dessert table on the cover—you'll drool all over the book. Instead, slip right back to page 306 where twenty-six pages of "Low-Calorie Gourmet Desserts" begin.

The first recipe hit me right in the tummy—"Low-Calorie Apple-Cheese Cake." My two favorite things in the whole world are apple pie and cheese cake, and here they were combined. A stroke of culinary brilliance. The recipe makes eight servings and each serving has only 128 calories.

There are also directions on how to make Low-Calorie Banana Cream Pie (half the calories of regular banana cream pie), Low-Calorie Walnut Torte (88 calories), and Low-Calorie Chocolate Nut Brownies (makes 32 brownies at only 55 calories each). (But whoever heard of eating only one brownie?)

All the recipes come from "Dominique's," one of Washington, D.C.'s, most outstanding French restaurants. By the looks of slim Dominique in the cover picture, he stays with his own low-calorie desserts.

FIRE ISLAND COOK BOOK
by Georgiana M. Hull
$1.45 Paperback 127 pages
   Cornerstone Library

Fire Island is a resort island down the road quite a piece from New York. It's off the southern coast of Long Island between the Atlantic Ocean and the Great South Bay. Only thirty-five miles long and a couple of miles wide at the widest point, it's famous for sun, surf, and sex, not necessarily in that order.

I was part of a "grouper" house there for three years. The sun and the surf were terrific. Other than that, all I can vouch for is the fish, which brings me back to *The Fire Island Cook Book*. I've included it in this catalog because it has some sensational fish recipes you can

use—and we all know that fish is one of the lowest-calorie, highest-protein foods available. Fish is very big on Fire Island because it's caught fresh every day. There are lots of low-calorie recipes—by famous food editors and gourmets such as Craig Claiborne, Alice Petersen, Geraldine Rhoads, Silas Spitzer, and Euell Gibbons—for clams, scallops, mussels, striped bass, bluefish, snappers, and eel. Just be cautious when a recipe calls for oils and sugar.

AMERICA'S BEST VEGETABLE
   RECIPES
by the Food Editors of *Farm Journal*
$6.95 Hardbound 336 pages
   Doubleday

Anything done by the Food Editors of *Farm Journal* sounds very authentic and down-home, and one look at this book conjures up visions of a robust, rosy-cheeked farm woman in a calico dress bustling about in a kitchen just a few feet away from the vegetable garden. Actually, I've never been hot for vegetables. The only nonfattening vegetables I like are carrots. They're crunchy, low-calorie, and take a long time to eat because they get stuck in your teeth. Naturally, I love all kinds of potatoes, corn on the cob dripping with butter, and salads loaded with cheese dressing. But with 666 different recipes in this book, you can pick out any number of delicious-sounding low-calorie vegetable recipes for such dishes as Blue Devil Onions, Marinated Mushrooms, Wax Bean Chowder with Bacon, Egyptian Okra-Beef Dinner, Hot Spiced Beets, and Farmhouse Green Salad with Garlic Dressing.

The chapter titles give you a fuller idea of what's in the book: "Garden Fresh Vegetables"; "Frozen Vegetables"; "Canned Vegetables"; "Dried Vegetables"; "Mixed Vegetables"; Vegetable Main Dishes"; "Vegetable Salads"; "Vegetable Soups, Seasonings, Sauces and Salad Dressings"; "Appetizers and Relishes"; and "Freezing and Canning Vegetables."

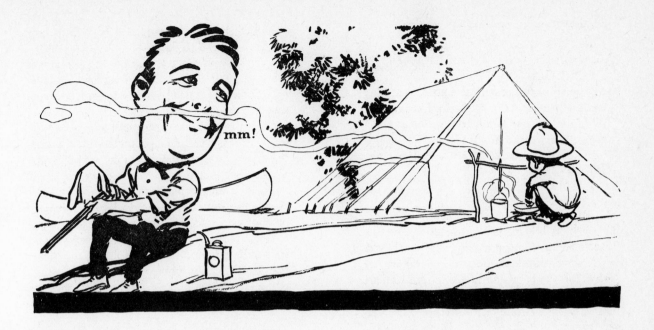

THE MICROWAVE OVEN COOKBOOK
by Loyta Wooding
**$1.95 Paperback 291 pages Pocket
Books**

The big reason why I'm including a microwave cookbook in a diet catalog is that I'm sneaky. See, microwave cooking is so fast, you're not going to have time to rummage around the refrigerator looking for a little something like that new sour cream cheese dip or an old piece of cherry pie on the second shelf while you're waiting for dinner to be done.

There are other reasons, too. You don't need oil or fat to cook with, and when cooking low-calorie vegetables you won't lose a lot of nutrients as you would if you cooked them in water on top of the stove.

After a preliminary thirty-page discussion of the hows and why of the whole microwave phenomenon, the author lists over 300 recipes and menus—a lot are fattening but there are plenty that are low-calorie, like a little number called Baked Chicken of the Islands, which uses a three-pound broiling chicken, a cup of unsweetened pineapple juice, and a lot of spices. The whole bird takes only twenty minutes to cook and it sounds delicious. Can't beat that for speed and yumminess.

THE OFFICE COOKBOOK
by Jody Cameron Malis
**95¢ Paperback 157 pages Pocket
Books**

Tired of spending all that money for lunch? Tired of being pushed and shoved so that someone else can have your seat? *The Office Cookbook* is about preparing your lunch right in the office so you don't have to put up with all that jazz. And it saves you money to boot.

There is a small diet section in the book with diet do's and don'ts and a list of special "urge fighting" foods to keep on the premises. That way you won't succumb to the doughnuts on the coffee wagon.

Sixteen "super low-calorie menus" give you the recipes for such lunches as "Office Vitality Booster," "Take-It or Leave-It Salad," and the "Sweetheart Plate: half cantaloupe filled with diced fresh fruit; Orange Sherbet; slice date nut bread—(225 calories)." Fortunately for those of us without a hotplate or stove in our offices, the Sweetheart Plate, like most of the recipes in this book, does not require any actual cooking.

THE AMERICAN HEART ASSOCIATION COOKBOOK
Recipes selected, compiled and tested under the direction of Ruthe Eshleman and Mary Winston, Nutritionists of the American Heart Association
$2.25 Paperback 403 pages Ballantine Books

The American Heart Association wants you to cut down on fatty foods because too much fatty food can be damaging to the heart and blood vessel system. As they point out, "Dietary intake of fat is only one of the factors linked with the catastrophic rise in heart and blood vessel diseases. But it is one factor that we ourselves can do something about." They also say,

"Overweight may bring a high risk of cardiovascular disease."

This is not really a diet book, although it does give the calories for each recipe. It is a cookbook for people who like to cook and eat whether they're young or old.

The hundreds of recipes have been selected from thousands submitted by friends, volunteers, and nutritionists of the A.H.A. from across the country.

There are sections on appetizers, soups, meats, fish, poultry, and desserts, plus advice on shopping, cooking, and adapting your own recipes. You can dine on such salivary superstars as Ratatouille, Steaks Brazilian, Crab Meat Maryland, and Raspberry Chiffon Pie, secure in the knowledge that $2.25 is a small price to pay for a lot of life insurance.

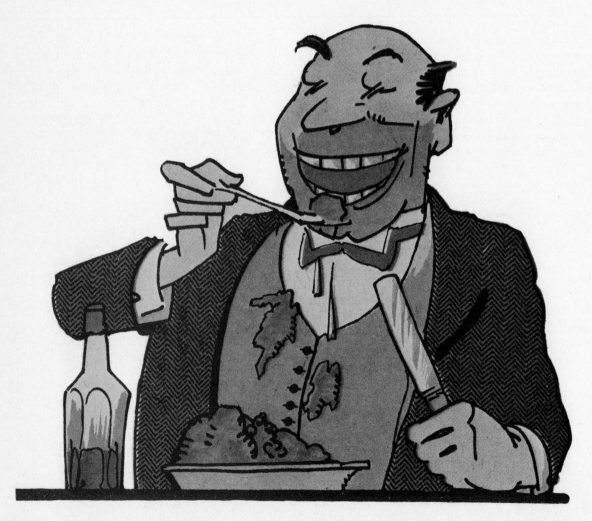

DIET FOR A HAPPY HEART
by Jeanne Hones
$7.95 Hardcover; $4.95 Paperback
192 pages 101 Productions

In *Diet for a Happy Heart* the author has created or adapted 200 recipes for a low-cholesterol, low-saturated-fat, sugar-free diet that includes such continental jazz as *coq au vin,* veal parmigiana, cold caviar soup, and low-cholesterol soufflés.

This book lists not only the calories per portion of these recipes, but also the cholesterol count. And there's a list of 300 foods with their calorie, cholesterol, protein, carbohydrate, and fat contents.

Beautifully illustrated, *Diet for a Happy Heart* would make a thoughtful gift.

THE SALT-FREE DIET COOKBOOK
by Emil G. Conason, M.D., and Ella Metz,
    Dietician
**$1.95 Paperback 143 pages Grosset
and Dunlap**

For anyone suffering from hypertension—or indeed anyone who must watch his or her salt intake—a doctor and a dietician have developed a cookbook with 150 recipes and menus to add variety and zest to breakfast, lunch, and dinner.

There are 1200-calorie menus for weight reducers and a salt-free diet for diabetics. Eating out? The authors tell you what to order and give you sample menus.

Each recipe and menu also has its sodium and calorie counts. Furthermore, 600 essential foods are listed with the salt content of each.

"How mightily sometimes
we make comforts of our losses."
ACT IV, SCENE 3
All's Well That Ends Well

"O Bottom, thou art changed!"
ACT III, SCENE I
A Midsummer Night's Dream

"All losses are restored."

NO. XXX
Sonnets

THE LOW BLOOD SUGAR COOKBOOK
by Margo Blevin and Geri Ginder
Foreword by Herbert B. Goldman, M.D.
$8.95 Hardbound 520 pages
   Doubleday

As the jacket of this book says, "If you can't eat sugar, potatoes, rice, bread, wheat, corn, some fruits and most prepared foods, what can you eat?"

That's a very good question, and the purpose of this book is to give those people who have low blood sugar, or hypoglycemia, over 800 sugar-free recipes so they won't have to live the rest of their life eating broiled steaks and tossed salads.

But people who *don't* have low blood sugar can also benefit from the 150 dessert recipes, unusual and enticing vegetable recipes, and carefully adapted Chinese, Italian, Jewish, and Mexican recipes with protein added and sugar and starches removed.

The Low Blood Sugar Cookbook is an encyclopedia of information about hypoglycemia,

and it *can* be a help in your losing weight. But be careful, O chubby one: some of the recipes can be high-calorie. Read everything very carefully.

COOKING WITHOUT A GRAIN OF SALT
by Elma W. Bagg
$6.95 Hardbound 224 pages
   Doubleday

Cooking Without a Grain of Salt contains over 250 low-sodium recipes. Each recipe tells you the exact sodium content in milligrams, as well as giving specific calorie-counts for each dish. There are suggestions for maintaining the low-sodium count while traveling, dining out, and visiting friends. Also included are foods to be generally avoided and information on how to use herbs, spices, seasonings, and flavorings.

This is an invaluable book for those who must eliminate salt from their diet, but don't want to be condemned to a life of bland, tasteless food.

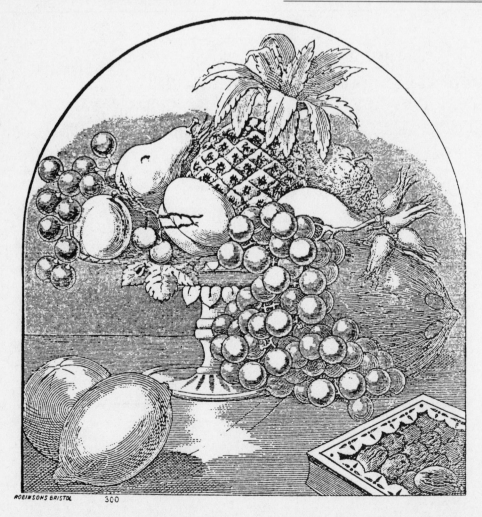

ROBINSONS BRISTOL   300

DIABETIC MENUS, MEALS AND RECIPES
by Betty M. West
Introduction by Russel F. Rypins, M.D.
$6.95 Hardbound 254 pages
Doubleday

You know how diabetics must watch their weight, sugar intake, and calories. Well, in this book there are menus and recipes for fourteen days of breakfasts, lunches, and dinners made up of a wide variety of foods. Each menu food is broken down into weight by grams and into amounts of carbohydrates, proteins, fats, and calories. There are also totals of the above for each meal.

The recipe section covers everything from soups to desserts. Each of the recipes is also broken down into grams of carbohydrates, proteins, fats, and calories. Some are even broken down into the food values of individual portions.

There are many, many recipes for such delectables as Ham Mousse (174 calories per serving), Golden Orange Salad (29 calories per serving), and Whipped Cocoa Cream (98 calories per serving).

This book first came out in 1949 but has recently been revised. I imagine if people are still using *Diabetic Menus, Meals and Recipes* after twenty-eight years, it must work.

ENJOYING FOOD ON A DIABETIC DIET
by Edith M. Meyer
$2.95 Paperback 227 Pages Dolphin Books

Flat out I'm going to tell you that this is a terrific cookbook, in my not-so-humble opinion. The title is not so hot, but the writing is funny and personal, the recipes sound delicious, nutritious, and low-calorie, and the whole thing is loaded with information.

The book differs from other diabetic cookbooks in that it is aimed at the "mild diabetic" who doesn't need to take insulin. Edith Meyer is herself a mild diabetic and has developed over 200 gourmet recipes that can allow the mild diabetic or those with overweight or heart problems to eat like a human being and still lose weight.

There are exchange lists of foods that are easy to figure out, and each recipe gives you total calories too. Your lips will quiver at the recipes for Astounding Standing Rib Roast, Oriental Adventure Salad, and Really Chocolate Tapioca Pudding (165 calories). And since the recipes are low in calories, they're good for anyone who wants to lose weight.

THE CALCULATING COOK:
A GOURMET COOKBOOK FOR DIABETICS & DIETERS
by Jeanne Jones
$6.95 Hardbound; $4.95 Paperback
192 pages 101 Productions

In 1975, *The Calculating Cook* was approved by the American Diabetes Association for use by diabetics.

The author, a diabetic herself, believes that being on a restricted diet should not limit the fun of eating. So she invented "whipped cream" toppings without cream, jams without sugar, and hollandaise sauce with only two tablespoons of butter.

The Calculating Cook translates practically every known food into food exchange values and gives exact calorie and exchange counts for individual servings of the recipes included. The book also has seventy sample menus for diets ranging from 800 to 3000 calories per day. This is a boon not only for diabetics, but for any of us wishing to control our weight.

References and Sourcebooks

Remember that chicken wing you licked clean for dinner? Do you want to know how many calories, vitamins, or grams of fiber it contained? Are you curious about whether it contained anything healthful—or harmful? Well, you can curl up with any of these books by the hour and get yourself an education in nutrition.

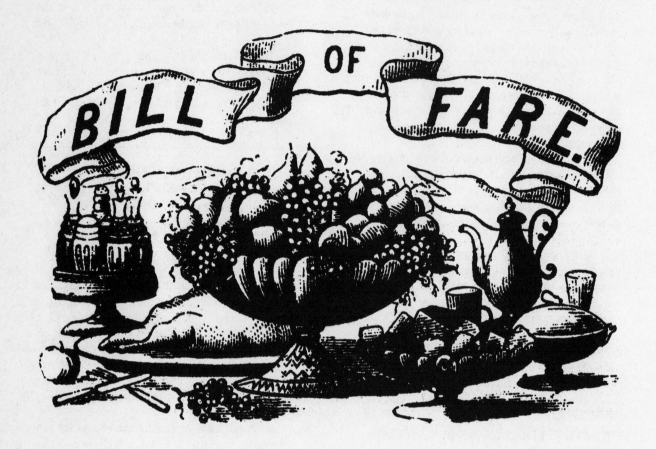

This section is devoted to those reference books which will give you a thorough analysis of most anything you'll ever eat. The one I use the most is the brand-name calorie-counter. Even if the author doesn't have your particular brand listed, you can still estimate the correct calorie count by finding a similar food. Just be sure the weights are the same.

Your diet education is never complete. Everything you learn can be a plus in your fight against the demon calorie, and for good health. You'll find something of value in all these books, and will probably end up wondering how you ever lived without them.

THE BRAND NAME FOOD GAME CONSUMER GUIDE
$1.95 Paperback 385 pages Signet Books

All of you are familiar with *Consumer Guide,* the magazine that rates everything and carries no advertising. Now they've compiled a book of thousands of brand-name foods and broken them down according to calories, carbohydrates, protein, fat, sodium, iron, and Vitamin A, Vitamin C, thiamin, riboflavin, and niacin. You can find out which brand-name foods are high in vitamins and minerals, but low in carbohydrates, which foods are best for a low-sodium diet, and which brand-name foods meet your diet requirements.

For instance, Swanson Hungry Man Frozen Boneless Chicken Dinner weighs 19 ounces; it contains 770 calories, 69 grams of carbohydrate, 43 grams of protein, 35 grams of fat, 2180 milligrams of sodium, 20 percent iron, 8 percent Vitamin A, no Vitamin C, 20 percent thiamin, 20 percent riboflavin, and 70 percent niacin.

There's a long introduction with discussions and explanations of the new federal labeling law, how to read the labels, food dating and what the government recommends as your daily vitamin requirements. There's even a discussion of private labels.

I've always been a freak for curling up with charts, and this is one of the best to curl up with. Now all of you—dieters and nondieters alike—can jump into bed, get under the covers, and find out everything you ever wanted to know about Weight Watchers Frozen Flounder Dinner.

THE BRAND-NAME CALORIE COUNTER
by Corinne Netzer with Elaine Chaback
$1.50 Paperback 188 pages Dell Books

What a job. There are 5000 brand-name listings: "a dieter's guide to the supermarket!" And that it is. I've used it for five years and found it indispensable, since it covers almost every brand-name food product you can think of. The ones that are missed you can estimate yourself to within a few calories, because in every category there will be a similar brand-name product.

Some examples: Swanson's three-course, 16-ounce fried chicken TV dinner, 652 calories; Budweiser beer, an 8-ounce glass, 105 calories; Hostess Twinkies, one ⅜-ounce cake, 133 calories.

My *Brand-Name Calorie Counter* pages are all wrinkled, because I read the book and weep at the calories of my favorite foods.

THE DIETER'S CHECKLIST
by E. W. Smith, Jr.
$1.45 Paperback 160 pages Dolphin Books

The Dieter's Checklist is one of those diet books loaded with all kinds of tables. You can have a big time checking everything out and maybe roll around on the floor with a pencil figuring out what exactly was in that lobster you just knocked off.

The book gives you your recommended daily requirements for minerals, vitamins, amino acids, cholesterol, and fatty acids. It also breaks many foods down into calories, carbohydrates, proteins and fats. There are also plenty of blank tables, so you can list everything you ate and how healthy and nutritious it was.

If you're a numbers freak, this is more fun than a warm glazed doughnut. As for me, I panic just trying to balance my checkbook.

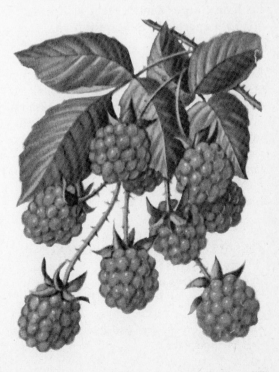

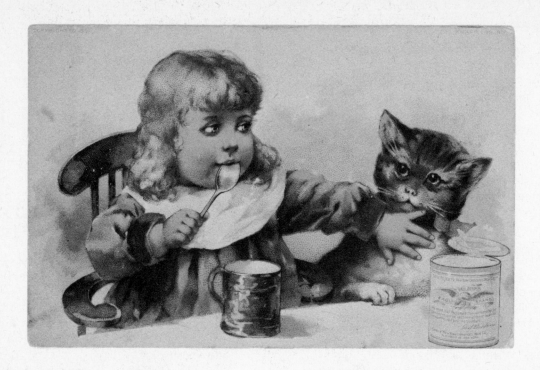

You diet folks are truly going to have a good time with these next five books. Take them down on the rug. Open them to any page and figure, calculate, and amaze yourself on how much information you find. You may want to buy an IBM computer to help you. Or get your wife, husband, lover, or what-have-you and read responsively on muggy afternoons.

THE ALL-IN-ONE CALORIE COUNTER
by Jean Carper and Patricia A. Krause
$1.50 Paperback Bantam Books

You can get your teeth into 5500 entries here. Look at some of the exotic classifications: chewing gum. (Juicy Fruit has 9.4 calories), Chinese food, blintzes, and yogurt. The listings also include low-calorie foods, health foods, fresh foods, and brand-name foods. I've been reading calorie-counters for years and I always learn a little something new. For instance, from this book, I just learned that seventeen French fries have 153 calories. Damn.

THE ALL-IN-ONE CARBOHYDRATE
GRAM COUNTER
by Jean Carper and Patricia A. Kraus
$1.50 Paperback Bantam Books

This is the one for all you low-carbohydrate dieters. Again there are 5500 listings (I think these authors like that number) with brand names, fresh foods, and health foods. If you're on a low-carbohydrate diet you should keep this book in your jeans. It's indispensable. Where else would you learn that four ounces of Grosse & Blackwell canned plum pudding has 62.4 grams of carbohydrate? That's a whole day's ration on some low-carbohydrate diets.

Other interesting tallies are: one seven-ounce can of Chicken of the Sea tuna, packed in oil, no carbohydrates; one small jar of Heinz baby food peaches, 37.9 grams of carbohydrates; one can of Gerber's orange-apple-banana juice, 20.1 grams of carbohydrates. A lot of carbohydrates in baby foods.

THE BRAND NAME NUTRITION
COUNTER
by Jean Carper
$1.95 Paperback Bantam Books

Get a couple of dollars out from under the mattress and go buy The Brand Name Nutrition Counter. This book is a gold mine of information, with over 2500 brand-name products and basic foods rated for vitamin, calorie, and carbohydrate content. It should help you with any diet you might go on. You'll find out what are super foods, what are junk foods, how much salt, carbohydrate, fat, calories, protein, Vitamin A, Vitamin C, Vitamins B–1 and B–2, niacin, and calcium foods contain. Again, this is a very important diet book.

THE ESSENTIAL VITAMIN COUNTER
by Martin Ebon
$1.75 Paperback Bantam Books

Mr. Ebon has alphabetically listed 1100 foods and their vitamin contents, as given by the U.S. government. There are no calorie or carbohydrate counts. Dieters can use the book to tell what kind of nutrients they're getting for their calories. Each section, such as "Dairy Products," has an informative and easy-to-read preface, and tells what kind of food preparation retains the most natural vitamins and how to read the new U.S. RDA vitamin information on food labels.

THE BARBARA KRAUS GUIDE TO FIBER IN FOODS
$1.50 Paperback 204 pages Signet Books

Everyone must know by now the latest development in nutrition, the high-fiber diet. According to some gurus in the medical profession, everything suggests that a high-fiber diet can help prevent such diseases as cancer of the colon and rectum, heart disease, diverticulosis, appendicitis, gallstones, varicose veins, hiatus hernia, hemorrhoids, and obesity. High fiber can also help relieve constipation and will lower serum cholesterol in the body.

In *The Barbara Kraus Guide to Fiber in Foods,* she provides the best available information on the fiber and calorie content of thousands of foods, both basic and brand-name.

For instance, Kellogg's All-Bran has 2.4 grams of fiber per ounce, while half a grapefruit from California or Arizona has 0.2 grams of fiber.

If you're a high-fiber freak like I am, this book will stay close to your heart or another part of your anatomy.

You may have noticed that a lot of food substitutes or supplements include Vitamin B–6 pills—which leads one to wonder whether we all shouldn't take extra vitamins if we're on a diet. If you wonder about this, there's a brochure called "Vitamins," available from Lederle Laboratories Division, Pearl River, New York 10965, which is six pages of everything you always wanted to know about vitamins but were afraid to ask. For instance, did you know that the word "limey" came from the 1800s when British sailors started eating limes to avoid scurvy? Or that the word *vitamin* came from a young researcher named Casimir Funk in the early part of the twentieth century?

The purpose of the brochure is to tell us that even in America today there is much vitamin deficiency. In 1969 a White House Conference on Food, Nutrition, and Health reported that while some fifty million Americans consume too many calories, twenty million are malnourished.

Quoting from page 5: "There appears to be a need for a balanced supply of all these vitamins and other essential nutrients to insure complete well-being, not just absence of disease. This is especially true in times of stress; the rapid growth of the young years, the critical months of pregnancy, the trying times of strict dieting for the overweight, the senior years, when many elderly people find their appetites fading. For many of these people, vitamin supplements can supply the nutrients that food does not."

Page 6 is a gold mine. It lists all the recommended daily allowances as recommended by the U.S. government and tells exactly what you have to eat to get these vitamins.

I asked my doctor once if I should take a vitamin supplement. He said in his Groucho Marx imitation, "Sure, if you want the most expensive urine in New York." But doctors differ. I think mine is a faith healer.

"A full belly makes a dull brain."
—Benjamin Franklin

THE BARBARA KRAUS DICTIONARY OF PROTEIN
$1.95 Paperback 345 pages Signet Books

This is a valuable sourcebook for whatever diet (or budget) you're following, since it gives the protein content per serving for practically everything edible. There are thousands and thousands of brand names and basic foods listed and the number of calories for each listing is also included.

You'll find out that you don't have to rely only on animal products to get your protein. You can eat all kinds of vegetables, grains, and nuts to get your valuable protein.

Whether you're a calorie-counter or a vegetarian, you can find the protein quotient of everything from almonds to zucchini and from soybeans to pizza.

CALORIES AND CARBOHYDRATES
by Barbara Kraus
$1.95 Paperback 370 pages Signet Books

Barbara Kraus is the *Encyclopedia Britannica* of the diet- and health-book world. Every time I stroll through a diet-book section there's a new Barbara Kraus there—and I always pick it up and read for ten minutes.

In this volume, she lists over 8000 brand-name and basic foods with their caloric and carbohydrate counts. She lists the basic foods, from meat and fish to fruits, vegetables, and grains, and brand-name products—McDonald's, Campbell's, Birds Eye, Celeste, Sunshine, Jeno's, Betty Crocker, Weight Watchers, and many more. What her books do is take the guesswork out of dieting.

Betcha I know what you wanted to ask when you saw "McDonald's" on the list. Okay, here it is. A Big Mac has 561 calories and 42.2 grams of carbohydrate. Don't get nervous. If you eat only one, you can still fit under the golden arch.

Note: In the 1976 edition this sourcebook was split into two volumes, *The Barbara Kraus 1976 Calorie Guide* and *The Barbara Kraus 1976 Carbohydrate Guide,* both published (as before) by Signet Books, both $1.25, and both as good and informative as ever.

THE DICTIONARY OF SODIUM, FATS AND CHOLESTEROL
by Barbara Kraus
$3.95 Paperback 366 pages Grosset & Dunlap

This is a one hefty book, but don't be intimidated—it's a major source of invaluable information regardless of what kind of diet you're on. You can instantly calculate the sodium, fat, and cholesterol content of everything you eat. It takes the guesswork out of healthful meal-planning.

Each of over 9000 brand-name and basic foods is broken down into the amount of sodium, saturated and unsaturated fats, and cholesterol each contains.

For instance, one ounce of Pringle's Potato Chips has 255 milligrams of sodium, 3 grams of saturated fat, 7 grams of unsaturated fat, and no cholesterol. The book also gives you the source of information—whether it's the U.S. Department of Agriculture or the manufacturer.

Get a small wagon, go to your local book store and drag it home. It's worth it.

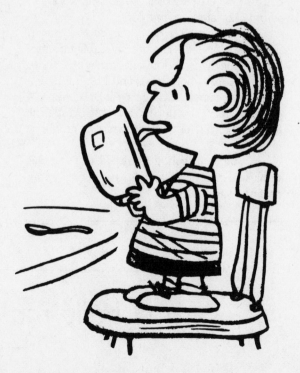

Pamphlets and Booklets, Cheapies and Freebies

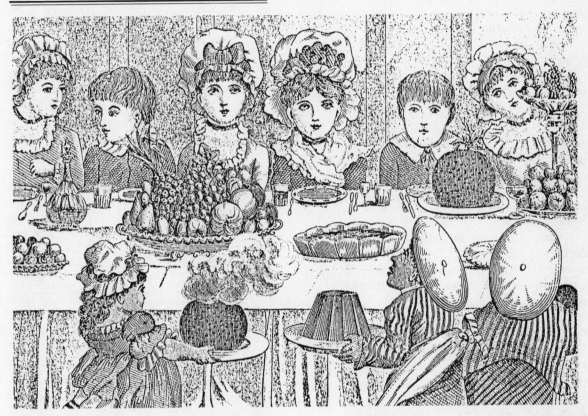

Our government is a gold mine of diet information. Mainly because your gold and mine are paying for it all. There's loads of information available on dieting, nutrition, and calorie-counting. I've described some of the booklets available; to see the complete listing, send for the free catalog (see page 82), and for a few dollars you can then order a whole stack of publications on weight reduction.

There is also a wealth of cheap paperbacks available—some are condensations that cost about a third or half as much as the originals, others are pamphlets put out by some company or other as a promotion or a public service. I like them because they're easy and fast to read. These little books can be found almost everywhere: dime stores, drugstores, and newsstands, or write to the publisher.

The only diet information that's better than cheap is free. Just because it doesn't cost anything doesn't mean it isn't worth anything. Many of the free goods available are terrific—in many ways, better than some of the diet information you have to buy.

The companies and associations that I list here have dieticians, statisticians, nutritionists, home economists, and God knows who all else working on getting weight-reducing news to you. Sure, they're pushing their insurance and products, but who cares? The price is right, their self-interest and yours often overlap (especially in the case of the insurance companies, obviously), and the publications are yours for the asking. So ask.

Cheapies

"YOU CAN REDUCE," published by the National Live Stock and Meat Board
36 South Wabash Avenue
Chicago, Illinois 60611
30¢   32 pages

"You Can Reduce" is an excellent diet pamphlet. Of course, the emphasis is on the consumption of meat in your diet, but the diet itself is nutritionally sound as well as effective. It makes several suggestions that I've never seen in a weight-reduction book. Maybe some of the following can work for you.

"Choose a Partner." Misery loves company; maybe you could lose weight with someone who's in the same boat. And there are enough of them around that finding one shouldn't be very difficult.

"Decide on a Date." Then be firm in your decision to get started. No more putting dieting off until tomorrow.

"Keep it a Secret, at Least at First." You may find it easier to stick to the diet if you don't tell anyone. Then let everyone be surprised when they suddenly notice your slimmer figure.

There are also ways to determine how many pounds you need to lose and how to find the best diet. You may choose from two low-calorie diets—a 1400-calorie diet and an 1800-calorie diet—depending on your physical activities. The booklet offers meal plans for the two diets, as well as a calorie chart and a column listing the grams of protein in various foods so that you can make your own meal plans.

The National Live Stock and Meat Board publishes other materials that could be of help:

"MEAT AND YOUR HEART"   15¢
12 pages
"YOU CAN REDUCE"   (pocket edition)
5¢   6 pages

Special Diet Series: These and other therapy-related publications are available only to professional people upon special request. Topics include weight reduction, high-protein/high-iron diets, diets for the diabetic, low-fiber diets, and sodium-restricted diets.

American Diabetes Association, Inc.
1 West 48th Street
New York, New York 10020

The American Diabetes Association feels there are several reasons for the tremendous increase in diabetes. One is improved health care and diagnosis. Another is that people are eating more and exercising less, and therefore becoming obese, which goes right along with diabetes. But the Diabetes Association says that most adult-type diabetes can be handled by diet alone.

They publish several booklets that could be of help to you. The cost is 20¢ each or three for 50¢. The number before the title indicates the number you should use when ordering.

101 "Canning Fruits without Sugar"
105 "Exercise, Calories and Diabetes"
137 "Statement on Saccharin"
144 "The Successful Treatment of Obesity"
147 "Nutrition: The Key to a Healthy Future"
156 "Health Foods"

The A.D.A. offers many more books and booklets than I've listed here. They will send you the complete list if you write them.

"EAT AND GROW SLIM"
Published by the American Institute of Baking
400 East Ontario Street, Chicago, Illinois 60611
25¢; money must accompany the order

"Eat and Grow Slim" has a straight-from-the-shoulder writing style that lays it right on the line for you. Like this quote: "The American Medical Association reports that you cannot rub off fat with massage, roll it off by machine, or boil it off in a steam bath. You must 'burn' it up by your own physical efforts."

The booklet offers a way to calculate your calorie quota, menus, a table of calories, and much more. Let me give you one more quote from the first page of the booklet; "Wishing that you might lose weight will make it so when your wishbone is supported by a firm backbone."

Special Menus Free!

for

Reducing   Constipation

Blood Building Weight Building

Acid Stomach Anemia

Diabetes   Auto-Intoxication

Given with Purchase
of

BATTLE CREEK
DIET SYSTEM
HEALTH FOODS
for Everybody

DANNON YOGURT
Dept. DC, 22–11 38th Avenue
Long Island City, New York 11101

Dannon Yogurt, the "no artificial anything" yogurt, publishes two booklets to help you lose weight.

"DIETING, YOGURT, AND COMMON SENSE"

This is a well-written booklet of forty-five pages. It starts with a hard-hitting introduction and covers such subjects as dieting and common sense, how you gain and lose weight, the value of exercise, and changing your eating habits.

They also offer two seven-day diets. One contains 900 to 1000 calories, the other 1500 to 1600 calories. This way you can vary the diets to suit yourself. Of course in both diets there is liberal use of Dannon yogurt. But Dannon explains: "You will note that these diets assign a primary role to yogurt. Of course, when Dannon recommends yogurt, our motives may be ulterior. But remember our cause is just. Yogurt contributes strongly to nutritional balance and we sincerely believe it makes sticking to a diet easier." There is also a seven-page calorie-counter. The booklet costs 25¢ to cover postage and handling.

"PLAIN YOGURT TASTE TREATS FOR PEOPLE WHO NEVER LIKED PLAIN YOGURT"

Just to make everything perfectly clear, plain yogurt has 150 calories per cup, flavored yogurts (coffee, lemon, vanilla) have 200 calories, and fruit yogurts have 260 calories. There are two lists in this four-page booklet; one lists sweet flavorings for plain yogurt, the other lists flavorings that are not sweet.

For example, the sweet list suggests adding one tablespoon liqueur. The nonsweet list suggests, for example, adding one teaspoon instant onion soup mix or other soup mix. Sounds good. Remember you have to use *plain* yogurt. This booklet is free.

"HOW TO LOSE WEIGHT AND LOVE IT"

by Dolly Reed Wageman
49¢
Carnation Company
DRW
3833 Eureka Drive
North Hollywood, California 91604

Being a bit of a male chauvinist, I got a little twitchy when I read this thirty-two-page booklet, because it's geared primarily toward women. But it has a lot of good diet ideas for men too, so I relaxed.

The booklet is published by the Carnation Company, and the diet is centered around their diet food, Slender.

Dolly Wageman, the author and former beauty editor of *McCall's,* sums it up best.

"What is the Slender Plan? This is a weight loss diet that combines Slender Diet Food for weight control from Carnation with low-calorie, conventional foods.

"How does the Plan work? On this diet you have six mini-meals a day! You eat something small and tasty every 2½ to 3 hours. This means you never go hungry."

Interspersed with the many menu plans are articles about improving your skin, face, and figure; there are exercises; and at the back of the book there are substitution lists of low-calorie foods and a weekly progress chart.

Ms. Wageman gives us fourteen different recipes for using Slender, with names like Orange Luscious, Slender Mocha Cocoa, and Slender Peaches 'N Cream. My personal favorite is Tangy Chocolate Shake. Mix one packet Dutch Chocolate Slender with six ounces nonfat milk and a quarter cup of chocolate yogurt. Only 204 calories, and yummy.

DIET WATCHER'S GUIDE

by Ann Gold and Sara Welles Briller
95¢ Paperback 155 pages Bantam Books

Diet Watchers are diet groups founded by one of the authors, Ann Gold. They are located in suburban New Jersey and suburban New York, which means if you live in Kalamazoo and want to follow the Diet Watcher's plan, you'll have to buy this book.

The keystone of this diet is the New York City Board of Health diet developed by Dr. Norman Jolliffe, but Gold and Briller have modified it to include some extras. And you don't need to count calories.

There are eight food groups in this diet:

Group 1 is unlimited foods. You can eat all you want of asparagus, cabbage, and pickles. Unlimited drinks include no-calorie soda pop, clear soups, and coffee and tea with no sugar or cream.

Group 2 is limited vegetables such as carrots, onions, and tomatoes. One serving of four ounces must be eaten every day.

Group 3 is fruits. You must eat three specified fruits every day, including one fruit high in Vitamin C.

Group 4 is meats, fish, and poultry. Fish must be eaten at least five times a week, and certain meats, fish, and poultry must be eaten three times a week.

Group 5 is bread. You must eat one slice of enriched white bread at breakfast and lunch every day.

Group 6 is eggs, which are limited to four to seven a week.

Group 7 is milk. You must drink two eight-ounce glasses of skim milk or buttermilk every day.

Group 8 is the list of "absolute don'ts." You should know this list by heart, from doughnuts to peanut butter. It's very important not to deviate from the basic Diet Watcher's diet with additions, subtractions, or substitutions.

Once you get to your desired weight you go on a maintenance program. It's to be hoped that while on the diet you have learned to eat the proper foods in a well-balanced way and that you have re-educated your "appestat"— the appetite regulator in your body. The authors hit you right in the breadbasket when they say, "Dieting is for a short time only, but maintenance is forever."

The *Diet Watcher's Guide* also has plenty of menus and recipes. The desserts look especially good. I'm going to try them myself, especially the Apple Malted: one apple, one cup skim milk, six thin ice cubes, and liquid nonsugar sweetener. You can substitute half a cup strawberries for the apple.

The authors say the diet can help you lose up to ten pounds the first week safely. Give it a try.

NEWSPAPERBOOKS
800 Third Avenue
New York, New York 10022

Dr. Jean Mayer was Professor of Nutrition at Harvard University when he wrote this book, and is now president of Tufts University. His column, "Food for Thought," is syndicated in over 100 newspapers throughout the country. The three books that I'm listing are among several that Dr. Mayer has written on food and nutrition, but these three deal primarily with weight control.

DR. JEAN MAYER'S 10 WAYS TO TAKE OFF POUNDS 50¢

This is a thirty-three-page booklet that has ten short chapters such as "Count Every Calorie," "Cook Lean Eat Lean," and "Exercise Off Calories." There's also a listing of 100-calorie portions of many foods.

DR. JEAN MAYER'S 31-DAY REDUCING DIET AND EXERCISE PLAN $1.50

Dr. Mayer outlines a whole month of diets, recipes, and exercises for you. For each day there is a 1200-calorie and a 1600-calorie diet. At the end of this eighty-page book there is a listing of foods and the time required to exercise off what you eat. Hold onto your pants for this one: "Boston Cream Pie, 1 serving 332 calories: To work off those 332 calories it takes 64 minutes of walking, 41 minutes of bicycling, 33 minutes of jogging, 30 minutes of swimming." After reading that, I dropped my fork as if it were a ton weight, with the meringue still on my teeth.

DR. JEAN MAYER'S LOW CALORIE FOODS FOR DIETERS WITH PORTION SIZES $1.25

This is a guide to a balanced, high-nutrition, low-calorie diet. There is a listing of 450 foods with portion sizes and their calories, plus some nutrition information.

I like Dr. Mayer's newspaper columns a lot and these books are just like the columns: clear, informative, and very helpful.

This isn't a book, but comes under the heading of "printed matter".

"THE SENSUAL DIETER'S GUIDE TO WEIGHT LOSS DURING SEX" Poster
At your poster store at varying prices.

Here it is: the real, the ultimate diet. The one you and I have been looking for. Of course the whole thing is a giggle, but I did hear once that an orgasm uses up about 1500 calories. My question is, does that count foreplay on a hot day?

Anyway, this is a poster that is about one by three feet. Since this catalog is not X-rated and is a book that I hope the whole family will use, I'll restrict myself to giving you only a few of the listings for calories supposedly burned up by various activities:

Fumbling Around   2 calories
Embracing and Hugging   5 calories
Anxiety   8 calories
Laughing   3½ calories

The rest you're going to have to read in the privacy of your boudoir.

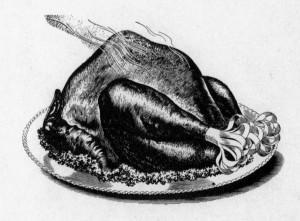

I've always had this thing for little books. For some crazy reason, I figure that the secret to the whole world of dieting could be held in the palm of my hand. Bantam Books has covered all the bases with a wide variety of small diet books. If you personally find the magic elixir, let me know immediately. Anyway, the books are cheap.

NATURAL FOOD DIETING
by Dina Boogaard   60¢

Learn why pure, unrefined foods are the best dietary basis for permanent weight loss. Which foods contain the health-giving nutrients you need to keep your weight low, your energy high. Sound, money-saving shopping advice. Health-giving helpful hints on preparing fruits, vegetables, grains, meats, fresh-from-nature foods. A natural-food starter diet with menus and easy-to-do recipes. And natural doesn't have to mean organic.

LOSE 7 POUNDS IN 7 DAYS
by Betsy Bliss $1.00

Betsy gives you 20 diets in 96 pages. It's a supermarket of crash diets. Pick your food—there's a crash diet to suit you: a grapefruit diet, a "Miracle" milkshake diet, a hotdog diet, and a six-meals-a-day diet. Whip off those seven pounds in seven days. (What happens the eighth day?)

FASTING: THE ULTIMATE DIET
by Allan Cott, M.D., with Jerome Agel and Eugene Boe $1.00

Dr. Cott put his fatter book on a diet and came up with this abridged edition. The cover says, "You may lose up to 5 pounds on a one-day fast and up to 10 pounds on a weekend fast." But before you start sewing your lips shut, remember, as Dr. Cott reminds you, to fast only with your doctor's permission and under his supervision.

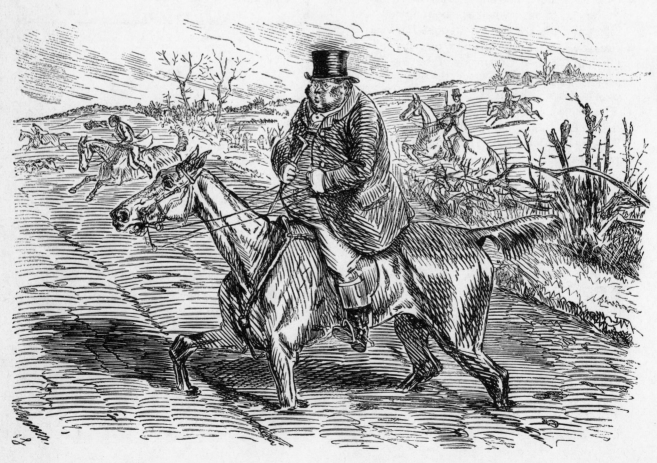

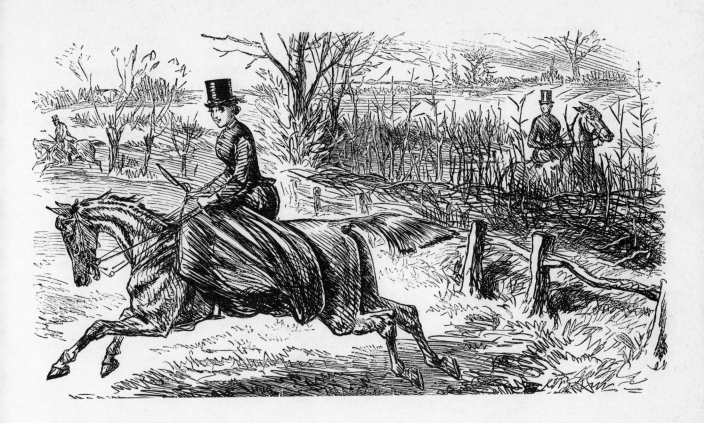

THE DIET HATER'S DIET BOOK AND GRAM COUNTER
by Joan Wexler 50¢

Stop counting calories—instead, cut carbohydrates (sugars and starches) to sixty grams daily and eat all the protein and fats (meat, fish, cheese, butter, and oil) you want. Ms. Wexler tried this one on herself, her husband, and three teenagers, and among them they lost fifty pounds.

THE NATURAL FIBER DIET
by Carter Chase $1.00

The magic of bran and natural fibers and how you can straighten out your whole eating life. According to the book, "This is the simple, inexpensive and tasty diet that keeps weight down as it helps protect you from six of the most serious diseases of civilization." Plus there are over forty delicious "natural fiber" recipes and special menus for dieters.

STOP DIETING! START LOSING
by Ruth West $1.00

It's a cookbook. It's a calorie-counter. It's a shopping guide. Ms. West says there are two basic ways to cut calories—one is to leave out high-calorie ingredients, the other is to substitute low-calorie ingredients for fattening ones.

She also tells you how to lose five pounds in two days and offers five sneaky tricks to keep you full.

NO-GUESS CARBOHYDRATE GRAM COUNTER
by Joan Wexler $1.00

Over 2500 exact carbohydrate gram counts including brand names, frozen foods, diet products, and low-carbohydrate snacks.

NO-GUESS CALORIE COUNTER
by Joan Wexler $1.00

Another of Ms. Wexler's valuable diet publications. This one gives thousands of exact, up-to-date calorie counts for all the foods you eat every day.

DIET WATCHERS GUIDE
by Ann Gold and Sara Wells Briller 60¢

An abridged edition of the original work (see above, page 70). The Diet Watcher Diet is used in the Diet Watchers' group located in New York and New Jersey. The basis of the diet is the New York City Health Department Diet.

THE SCALE-WATCHER'S DIET
by Evelyn Fiore
75¢ Paperback 190 pages Ace Books

The Scale-Watcher's Diet is a low-carbo-hydrate diet on which you are supposed to limit your daily consumption of "carbograms"—the amount of carbohydrates, measured in grams, contained in a food—to sixty. The foods that Evelyn Fiore tells us to look out for are: all baked goods, potatoes, pasta, breakfast cereals, dried fruits, and candy. There are other carbohydrate villains too, but these are the most obvious.

She also says on this diet we can lose ten, fifteen, or maybe even twenty pounds in thirty days.

In addition to the diet, Ms. Fiore gives us a fascinating history of the low-carbohydrate diet. The story is that in the 1860s a 5-foot 5-inch, 200-pound coffin-maker had an earache and went to the doctor. The doctor could find nothing wrong with his ear but thought that the problem was that fat was pressing on his eardrum. So he put him on a low-carbohydrate diet. The earache disappeared. He lost fifty pounds and cut his waistline by twelve inches at the end of one year. There's nothing better than a thin, happy coffin-maker.

One nice point for all elbow-benders—moderate drinking is okay.

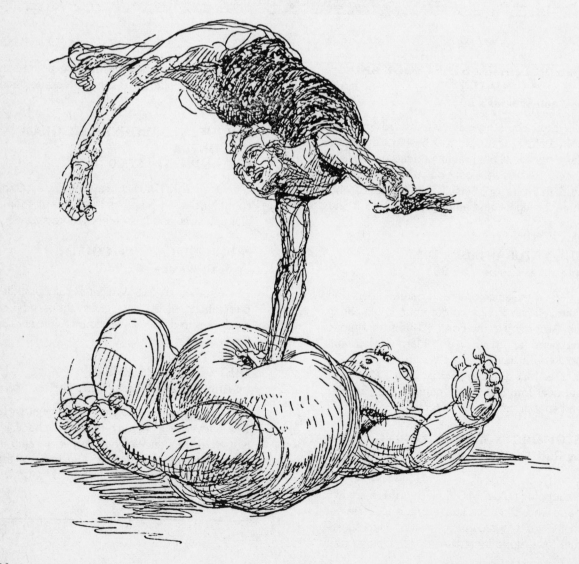

I can't eat just one piece of popcorn, and I can't buy just one of these little books. The Dell Purse Books are clear, concise, a good half-hour read, and they always make me think I'm going to discover the answer to all my dieting woes. This, of course, hasn't happened, but I still buy them all—at 35¢ apiece.

BRAND-NAME CARBOHYDRATE GRAM COUNTER

You don't count calories. You count carbohydrate grams, and simply limit your intake of sugars and starches to sixty grams a day.

BRAND-NAME CALORIE COUNTER

CARBOHYDRATE GRAM COUNTER

COUNT YOUR CALORIES

THE DOCTOR'S QUICK INCHES-OFF DIET

A quick synopsis of Dr. Stillman's larger paperback (see page 13).

THE DOCTOR'S QUICK WEIGHT LOSS DIET

Another synopsis of the original paperback title (page 13) by Dr. Stillman.

CELLULITE

Whatever that stuff is, this book tells you how you can supposedly get rid of it.

DIET TIPS & TRICKS

Many ideas, some extremely helpful. For instance: "Serve your food on smaller plates. Diet portions will appear less meager that way," "Go grocery shopping after you've eaten, never before," and "Start a neighborhood diet group." Who knows—if you're single you could meet someone nice.

THE TEN-DAY-10-POUND OFF DIET

Almost every gimmick diet from the Drinking Man's Diet to the Hotdog Diet and on through the Strawberry and Cream Diet. Seventeen different diets in all. (If *I* ate strawberries three times a day, I'd probably break out in such a rash that I'd look like a strawberry.)

FIVE DAY DIETS

For those who eat like crazy on the weekends and go cold turkey Monday through Friday. Many sample diet menus for that tough Monday-through-Friday time.

LOW-GRAM DIETS

THE TRUTH ABOUT WEIGHT CONTROL

An abridgement of Dr. Neil Solomon's book (see page 2). In this case I recommend that you spend the extra money and get the original. It's more complete, but this purse-size version is useful, too.

THE BOSTON POLICE DIET

THE COMPLETE CHOLESTEROL COUNTER

DR. STILLMAN'S 14 DAY SHAPE-UP

You know what this is (see page 13).

"The loss, the gain, the ordering on't, is all
Properly ours."

ACT II, SCENE I
A Winter's Tale

Freebies

"THE HEALTH WAY TO WEIGH LESS"
American Medical Association
Department of Foods and Nutrition
Copies of the pamphlet may be
purchased from the A.M.A. Order
Department OP-322
535 North Dearborn Street
Chicago, Illinois 60610

This is it. This is the straight poop from the guys who are supposed to know what it's all about when it comes to dieting.

In this pamphlet, the A.M.A. briefly gives you the basics of weight control plus answers to many of your questions. The booklet is only four pages long, but in that short space it manages to give you a mountain of information.

To me, two sections stand out. One is a formula for calculating your weight and calorie intake in order to subtract the correct number of calories you should consume in order to lose weight. The second section sums up what losing weight is all about, and does it better than I've ever seen elsewhere: "The only way to take in your belt or slip into that pantsuit again is to eat less and exercise more. But remember, no matter how much you huff and puff, you can't just shake it off, rock it off, roll it off, knock it off, or bake it off. An escapable exercise is turning your back on food and repeating many times a day the word 'no.' So, if you're going to diet, do it!"

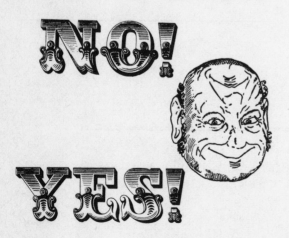

"FOOD & FITNESS"
Report by Blue Cross and Blue Shield of
Greater New York
622 Third Avenue
New York, New York 10017

Check with your local Blue Cross and Blue Shield office to see if they have the book. If not, write them at the above address or at their editorial offices at 840 North Lake Shore Drive, Chicago, Illinois 60611.

Blue Cross and Blue Shield went to some of the biggest names in the nutrition and exercise field to find authors for the articles in this booklet—people such as Frederick J. Stare, M.D., Jean Mayer, Ph.D., Joyce Brothers, Ph.D., astronaut James A. Lovell, and humorist Art Buchwald (who tells you his "Secret of Dieting").

"Food & Fitness" is loaded with goodies. There's a seven-day diet plan, "Food Fads," "Dollar-Wise Food Shopping," and "Getting Back in Shape," to name just a few.

NATIONAL RESEARCH COUNCIL
2101 Constitution Avenue, N.W.
Washington, D.C. 20037

"DIET AND CORONARY HEART DISEASE"
A Joint Statement of the Food and
Nutrition Board, Division of Biology
and Agriculture, National Academy of
Sciences–National Research Council,
and The Council on Foods and
Nutrition, American Medical
Association.

This is a three-page report published in July, 1972, on the relationship of diet and coronary heart disease. There are some scary facts for me and you to think about, such as "In 1970, for example, some 666,000 Americans, of whom about 171,000 were under the age of 65, died of coronary heart disease." There are certain "risk factors" that can be controlled, such as high-cholesterol levels, high blood pressure, heavy cigarette-smoking, obesity, and physical inactivity.

"VEGETARIAN DIETS"
A Statement of the Food and Nutrition Board Division of Biological Sciences Assembly of Life Sciences, National Research Council. Prepared by the Committee on Nutritional Misinformation.

This report was published in May 1974. Its purpose was to find out if a vegetarian diet could be nutritious. As the report says, "Most nutritionists agree that vegetarian diets can be adequate, if sufficient care is taken in planning them." The summary of the report states: "A vegetarian can be well nourished *if* he eats a variety of plant foods and gives attention to the critical nutrients mentioned above [in the report]. Dairy products and eggs are outstanding sources of the nutrients of greatest concern. Legumes, leafy vegetables, and a source of Vitamin B12 are important components of the diet containing no foods of animal origin."

METROPOLITAN LIFE
One Madison Avenue
New York, New York 10010
Check with your local office on this free booklet or write to the above address.

"FOUR STEPS TO WEIGHT CONTROL"

The four steps are on the first page:

1. See your doctor.
2. Set your weight goal.
3. Retrain your eating habits.
4. Be more active.

Those fourteen words really wrap up the weight-losing business, but we all know it's going to take more than fourteen words to do the job. This is a thirty-two-page, clearly written, and well-produced booklet. Each of the four steps is discussed in detail, and a general discussion of overweight is included. And of course, being a life insurance company, Met Life is concerned about heart attacks, so there is a section on the "Cholesterol Controversy," which points out that "it has not been proved that high cholesterol levels by themselves cause 'coronaries.'"

THE EQUITABLE LIFE ASSURANCE SOCIETY OF THE UNITED STATES
Box 580, General Post Office
New York, New York 10001
Check with your local office for this free booklet or write to the above address.

I've never seen so much information packed into such a small space. There are sections on why we should watch our weight, how we can control our weight, and what we should know about calories, plus a calorie-counter and a daily diary. According to this brochure, it takes 100 minutes of sitting to use up 100 calories. In other words, we ought to get off our rear ends and *move*.

THE PRUDENTIAL INSURANCE COMPANY OF AMERICA
Prudential Plaza
Newark, New Jersey 07101
Check with your local office on these free booklets or write to the above address.

The Prudential Health Series

"HOW TO EXTEND YOUR LIFE SPAN" by Dr. Paul Dudley White

A very important booklet for everyone. Written by a top cardiologist, this sixteen-page booklet is crammed with good information. It deals not only with losing weight, but also with the importance of exercise, the hazards of cigarette-smoking, stress, and the effects of coffee on your body. I found one sentence very frightening. "In a study . . . of 200 coronary heart disease cases, 193 were male and only seven were female." Watch out, guys!

"THERE'S MORE TO FOOD THAN EATING"

A discussion of proteins, carbohydrates, fats, vitamins, and minerals, and tips on how to buy food wisely.

"IT'S FUN TO BE HEALTHY"

Primarily for boys and girls of school age. Talks about foods for growing up, and about exercise, cleanliness, rest, and colds. The last line of the booklet sums up its positive attitude: "Yes, it's fun to be healthy."

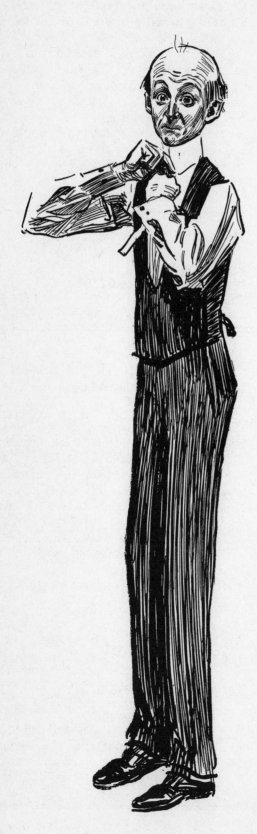

AMERICAN HEART ASSOCIATION
44 East 23rd Street
New York, New York 10010

The following booklets are all free from the American Heart Association, but I would check to see if they're available from your local Heart Association. If not, write the A.H.A. at the above address.

The American Heart Association is concerned primarily with fat control—that is, saturated fat—and offers a low-cholesterol plan to reduce the risk of heart attack.

The following booklets are available: "A Guide for Weight Reduction," "Save Food $$ and Help Your Heart," "The Way to a Man's Heart" (a fat-controlled, low-cholesterol meal plan to reduce the risk of heart attack), "Recipes for Fat-Controlled Low Cholesterol Meals," and "Healthy Eating for Teenagers."

These booklets are available only with a physician's prescription: "Planning Fat-Controlled Meals for 1200 and 1800 Calories," "Planning Fat-Controlled Meals for Approximately 2000-2600 Calories," "Your Mild Sodium-Restricted Diet," "Your 500 Milligram Sodium Diet," "Your 1000 Milligram Sodium Diet."

The booklets are short, easy to read, with lots of information—take them to heart.

THE ARTHRITIS FOUNDATION, INC.
New York Chapter
221 Park Avenue South
New York, New York 10003

The Arthritis Foundation publishes two free booklets on diet and arthritis. The titles are "Diet and Arthritis, A Handbook for Patients" and "The Truth about Diet and Arthritis."

As the first booklet points out: "Because overweight may put such a burden on your joints, usually causing greater inflammation and pain, you must face the possible need to get rid of damaging excess pounds. Your doctor, or the nutritionist or dietician to whom he refers you, is the best advisor on the diet you should follow."

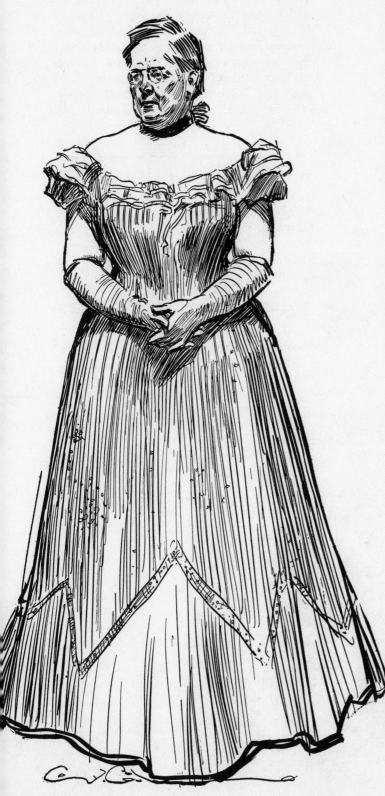

There is a great practical hint in "Diet and Arthritis": "As a basic guide, remember that foods LOW in calories are usually thin, dilute, clear, fresh, watery or crisp. Foods HIGH in calories are usually thick, oily, greasy, crisp, smooth, gooey, sweet or sticky, compact or concentrated, alcoholic."

"FACTS ABOUT OBESITY"

U.S. Department of Health, Education and Welfare
For sale by the Superintendent of Documents
U.S. Government Printing Office
Washington, D.C. 20402

This is a general survey of obesity that discusses obesity and health, the causes of overweight, motives for overeating, obesity in childhood and adolescence, consequences on obesity, and treatment of obesity. It covers two subjects not ordinarily discussed. First it gives a clear and concise explanation of the fat cell and its effect on overweight, which should be read by everyone.

Then it deals with the intestinal "bypass" surgery whereby the "ingested foods by-pass most of the small intestine where ordinarily, calories would be absorbed by the body." As the booklet points out, surgery should be done only when there is "massive obesity (when body weight is at least 100 pounds above or double the ideal weight)." The intestinal bypass operation is a last resort "when all other alternatives have failed to produce a lasting weight reduction, and when the complications of the obesity itself may be ultimately life-threatening."

Published by the United States Department of Commerce
National Oceanic and Atmospheric Administration
National Marine Fisheries Service
Washington, D.C. 20235

"SEAFOOD SLIMMERS"

"Seafood Slimmers" is a twenty-page, low-calorie fish recipe booklet that gives you scrumptious recipes and includes the calories per serving for each recipe. This book has been specially designed for the dieter and has, as an added plus, beautiful photographs of the fish you can prepare. Look at some of the recipes: Striped Bass with Low-Cal Stuffing (310 calories a serving); Spicy Snapper (130 calories a serving); Cantonese Shrimp and Beans (130 calories a serving); Chef's Salad Chesapeake (also 130 calories a serving). Enjoy yourself.

"SEAFOODS FOR HEALTH"

This booklet is exactly what it says. It tells you the nutritional characteristics of fish and shellfish, how you can custom-tailor diets with fish, how fish and shellfish can furnish many of the nutrients that are required by the body, how fish and shellfish are excellent sources of high-quality protein, the relationship of diet and heart disease, and more. "Seafoods for Health" also re-examines that old saw about fish being brain food. Allow me to quote from it: "Fish and a few other foods are often referred to by food faddists as brain food. There is no basis for this claim. In fact, no such thing as brain food exists, anymore than there is a big-toe food or a little-finger food." Son of a gun. I've been eating enough fish to grow fins. . . . no wonder I still don't know enough to come in from the rain.

"LET'S COOK FISH"

Now here's a terrific recipe book but it contains much more. Some of the sections cover nutritive value of fish, market forms of fresh and frozen fish, buying fish (including how much to buy, buying fresh fish, buying frozen fish, and buying canned fish), cleaning and dressing fish, storing and thawing fish, and how to cook fish. Let me warn you, this fifty-six-page booklet includes some very fattening ways to cook fish. Don't even look at such methods as deep-fat frying, oven-frying, and pan-frying. Instead, stick with baking, broiling, charcoal broiling (yummy), poaching, and steaming.

THE AMERICAN DIETETIC ASSOCIATION
430 North Michigan Avenue
Chicago, Illinois 60611

The following is a list of information kits and nutrition booklets available to the public.

"WEIGHT CONTROL" KT-0755 $1.50

This includes "A New Weigh of Life," "Food Facts Talk Back," "Position Paper on Nutrition Misinformation," a fact sheet for

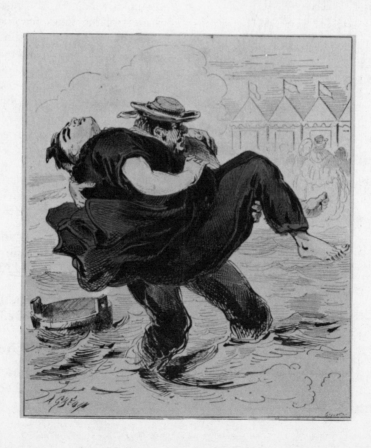

planning calorie-controlled meals, and an article on weight control by Frederick Stare.

"A NEW WEIGH OF LIFE" 1973
B0304 single copy free with stamped self-addressed long envelope

Two-color brochure, appealing to a general audience. Stresses the balancing of energy output with energy input from the four major food groups. Suggests food patterns and selection for weight loss and control.

"FOOD FACTS TALK BACK" B0301 75¢

A newly revised thirty-two-page booklet that discusses major food fallacies, giving the facts. Has sections on additives, vegetarianism, weight reduction, pregnancy, and balanced diets.

"NUTRITION: WHAT'S IT ALL ABOUT?" B0302 single copy free with stamped self-addressed long envelope

This two-color brochure, revised in 1975, discusses the four basic food groups and the essential nutrients.

"MEAL TIME—HAPPY TIME" B0303 single copy free with stamped self-addressed long envelope

Another 1975 revision, dealing with nutritional needs of children between one and the teen years. Pointers to parents helpful in counseling.

"DIABETIC" KT-0751 $1.50

This includes "Meal Planning with Exchange Lists," American Diabetes Association source list, a bibliography on diabetes, a list of visual materials, and an ethnic-foods exchange list.

"MEAL PLANNING WITH EXCHANGE LISTS" B0550 40¢

A twenty-page booklet for the person with diabetes.

"ETHNIC/DIABETES" KT-0753 $1.50

This includes "Understanding Food Patterns in the U.S.A.," "Meal Planning with Exchange Lists," the Spanish Diabetic Diet, six diet plans (American, Jewish, "soul" food, Ita-

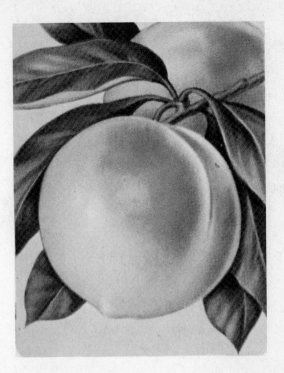

lian, Chinese, Mexican), and "Planning Ethnic Menus."

The American Dietetic Association also publishes many other booklets and kits and has films available. You may write them at the above address for their complete listings.

HOW TO LIVE WITH DIABETES
by Henry Dolger, M.D., and Bernard Seeman
Paperback 190 pages Pyramid Books
Distributed by the Upjohn Company
Kalamazoo, Michigan

This is a free book, available from the Upjohn Company, which will help the diabetic live with his condition on the best possible terms by providing him (or her), his family, and his friends with a full understanding of the disease.

I'll list the chapter titles so you can tell if this book is for you:

"What About Diabetes?" "Who Gets Diabetes?" "The Development of Diabetes," "The Search for a Cure," "Diet Diabetes," "The Meaning of Insulin," "Control with Insulin—The Tools," "Control with Insulin—The Techniques," "Orinase and the Oral Drugs," "The Complications of Diabetes," "The Diabetic Child," "The Diabetic Adolescent," "The Diabetic Adult," "Diabetes as a Special Problem for Women," and "From Today to Tomorrow."

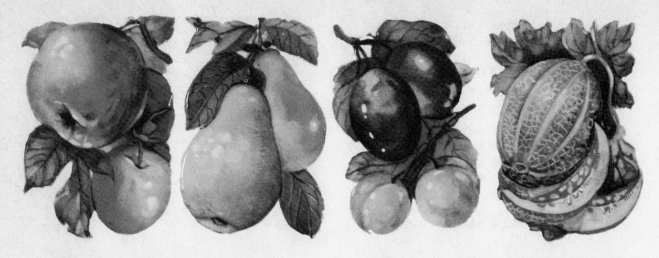

UNITED STATES DEPARTMENT OF AGRICULTURE
Office of Communication
Washington, D.C. 20250

Your friendly U.S. Department of Agriculture puts out a bunch of terrific food booklets and they're all free. I'll give you a short shot about each of them, even though some have nothing to do with losing weight. The fact is, these booklets are too good to miss, especially since your taxes pay for them. Besides, the food and nutrition information they contain is invaluable—and it's always fun to get a big package in the mail.

"FOOD AND YOUR WEIGHT"

A well-rounded (sorry) survey of food and your weight. There are discussions of your weight, daily calorie needs, basic weight control facts, tips for planning a day's food, suggestions for reducers, and calorie values of common foods. The authors have written a clear, concise, and excellent booklet—regardless of what diet you go on.

"FAMILY FARE—A GUIDE TO GOOD NUTRITION"

Another excellent source of food and cooking information. It gives you loads of solid nutrition information, tells how to buy food intelligently in your market and how to store and measure food, and gives recipes for meat, poultry, fish, eggs, cheese, vegetables, salads, soups, sauces, breads, sandwiches, and desserts. I found out from it that "oranges with a

slight greenish tinge may be just as ripe as fully colored ones." See what you can learn.

"EAT A GOOD BREAKFAST"

Breakfast and brunch have always been my favorite meals. (Come to think of it, lunch, dinner, and snacks aren't too bad either.) Anyway, this leaflet tells us the components of a good breakfast, how to have something different for breakfast, and the value of a good breakfast. Remember the adage: Eat breakfast like a king, lunch like a prince, and dinner like a pauper.

"FOOD GUIDE FOR OLDER FOLKS"

How the senior citizen can have good nutrition, including a discussion of the various food groups, how to save time and energy in cooking, how to use simple kitchen equipment, and many recipes. The main point of the booklet is that as we grow older, our needs for nutrients in food and food energy change. A valuable book for those getting up in years.

"NUTRITIVE VALUE OF FOODS"

A dynamite forty-two-page book giving the nutritive values of hundreds of foods. They break each food down into five different categories of vitamins, minerals, water, calories, and fat. And at the end of the book there is a table that tells you how much of each vitamin you should have, according to your age.

These are only a few of the booklets the Department of Agriculture publishes. Write for the complete catalog. If the others are anything like the ones I've just discussed, I'd get a copy of every one.

MEAD JOHNSON LABORATORIES
Evansville, Indiana

One of the continuing mysteries of my life is whether I need vitamins. My doctor says I don't. But the more I read and talk to people the more confused I get.

Anyway, this is a booklet from a company that manufactures vitamins. It gives a balanced viewpoint on when your children or you need vitamins. There is also a very helpful table at the end, listing the major vitamins, telling what they do for your body, and giving common food sources for them.

"CALORIE COUNTS"
Progresso Foods Corporation
100 Caven Point Road
Jersey City, New Jersey 07305

Calorie counts of many Progresso products. For instance, their minestrone soup has 100 calories per eight-ounce cup, while white clam sauce has 320 calories for the same eight ounces. Very useful for eaters of Progresso foods.

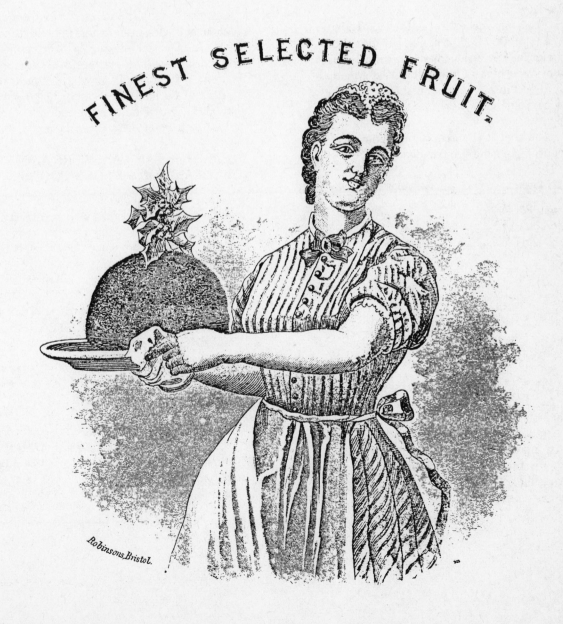

FINEST SELECTED FRUIT.

Robinsons Bristol.

**BEST FOODS CORPORATION
Dept. X, P.O. Box 307
Coventry, Connecticut 06238
All these booklets are free on a single
  copy basis.**

"A DIET FOR TODAY"

"A Diet for Today" has just entered the hallowed halls of the Goldberg Hall of Fame in Diet Literature. It's a wonderful diet book and a big bargain—it's free. It packs an amazing amount of weight-reducing and diet information into only thirty-two pages.

According to the book, "This diet seeks to alter your eating in four ways: it keeps cholesterol moderate to low; it lowers total fat consumed; it replaces some saturated fat with polyunsaturated and it keeps calories at a moderate level."

The daily menus in "A Diet for Today" come to around 2000 calories, which is about right for the average woman and should cause the average man to reduce his weight gradually. If you're a women you should probably reduce your calories to under 2000 to lose weight.

The diet itself breaks foods into seven groups. Here's the general idea:

Food Group	Servings Each Day
Protein Foods	2
Dairy Foods	2
Fruits and Vegetables	6 or more, including one high in Vitamin A, one high in Vitamin C
Breads, Cereal, Potato	4
Fats and Oils	4
Sugars, Syrups, Sweets	2
Desserts	2

"A Diet for Today" outlines seven days of sample menus and thirty recipes for dishes included in these menus. The advantage to the food group breakdown is that all the foods within a group have similar nutritional values, and are therefore interchangeable in the menus, thereby making menu-planning easier and more flexible.

"BEYOND DIET . . . EXERCISE YOUR WAY TO FITNESS AND HEART HEALTH"

The authors point out that the labor-saving machines and gadgets of the American lifestyle may seem to have improved life, but have actually shortened lives. All these conveniences have made us lazy. Our laziness has led to a lack of exercise, which, along with smoking, high blood pressure, and elevated blood cholesterol, leads to a much higher risk of heart attack. The booklet translates scientific principles into safe and realistic programs that can be followed by anyone. It warns against the pitfalls of an overenthusiastic launching of an exercise program, suggesting that you first see your doctor for a checkup.

"FOUR KEYS TO A HEALTHY HEART"

According to the authors, the four most influential and dangerous factors in heart disease are the food we eat (meaning a diet high in fats and cholesterol), high blood cholesterol, cigarette-smoking, and high blood pressure. This is an informative and entertaining booklet that gives you a new appreciation of your pumper and how to keep it healthy and happy.

"QUESTIONS AND ANSWERS ABOUT FATS AND OILS IN OUR FOODS"

In a few pages, you can get an education in fats and oils. Some of the slick questions answered are: What is the difference between fats and oils? What food values does fat have? What place does fat have in special diets? What information about fat can be found on labels of food products?

"GOOD RECIPES TO BRIGHTEN THE ALLERGY DIET"

Being your pal and one who has sneezed a lot, I threw this booklet in even if it isn't specifically a diet aid . . . although it could be. Depending on what you're allergic to, you can look up recipes which contain no wheat, no eggs, no milk, etc. So if you have to live within the limits of an allergy diet, this could be a big help. And on that note, I bid you a fond "achoo."

NUTRITION SERVICES
**General Foods Consumer Center
250 North Street
White Plains, New York 10625**

In addition to manufacturing diet food products, General Foods also publishes three booklets that could help you on your diet. Single copies are free.

"HERE'S THE WAY TO A SLIMMER LIFE"

This is an eight-page booklet that gives you a daily food guide, low-calorie garnishes, seasonings for salads, vegetables and entrées, certain dieting myths we've all heard about, and some helpful hints that can keep you on your diet.

"NEW TREATS FOR DIETERS"

This is a terrific recipe book using General Foods' D-Zerta products. For instance—get your fork poised—the first recipe in the book is for Dieter's Strawberry Cheesecake. One-sixteenth of the cake has only 81 calories and 4 grams of carbohydrates. You can't beat that.

"NUTRITION INFORMATION CAN WORK FOR YOU"

A valuable book that tells you what nutrition is and how to utilize nutrition labeling to help plan meals and provide adequate nutrition, and gives key nutrients, recommended daily allowances of twenty nutrients as recommended by the U.S. government, and nutrient values of all General Foods products on which nutrition labeling appears.

CEREAL INSTITUTE, INC.
**135 South LaSalle Street
Chicago, Illinois 60603**

"BE WISE! FOOD FACTS YOU SHOULD KNOW!"
"SEE THE FACTS ABOUT THE FOODS YOU EAT"

These are two free booklets put out by a national organization of the breakfast food industry. Obviously they are interested in getting you off to a good start with breakfast.

I've always subscribed to the old saying, "Eat breakfast like a king, lunch like a prince, and dinner like a pauper." Most nutritionists agree that you should have a nutritionally sound breakfast, because you're coming off a ten- to twelve-hour period without food.

If you eat a nutritious breakfast it will last you well into the afternoon. (That should stop us dieters from hitting the sweet rolls and a huge lunch.)

Breakfast cereals, either hot or cold, are convenient. And with the new labeling laws you can see the calories, proteins, carbohydrates, fats, and all the vitamins on each package.

One warning. Be careful of those presweetened cereals. They can be loaded with calories.

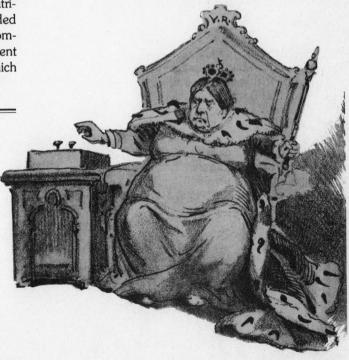

NABISCO, INC.
Consumer Services
East Hanover, New Jersey 07936

Nabisco publishes nutritional information on their leading products in kit form. The sheets in the kit are the size of your recipe file, which makes for easy reference.

Each product is on an individual sheet that shows the number of calories and the grams of protein, carbohydrate, and fat for an average serving as well as the percentages of the U.S. Recommended Daily Allowances for protein, vitamins, and minerals.

Let me give you a few examples: Barnum's Animal Crackers, one of my old favorites, have 130 calories in eleven crackers; two Fig Newtons have 23 grams of carbohydrates; one ounce of Nabisco 100% Bran Cereal with half a cup whole milk has 10 percent of the protein needed per day, as recommended by the government.

Send in for this kit and find out exactly what's in the Nabisco products you've been eating.

TWO

THE INNER PERSON

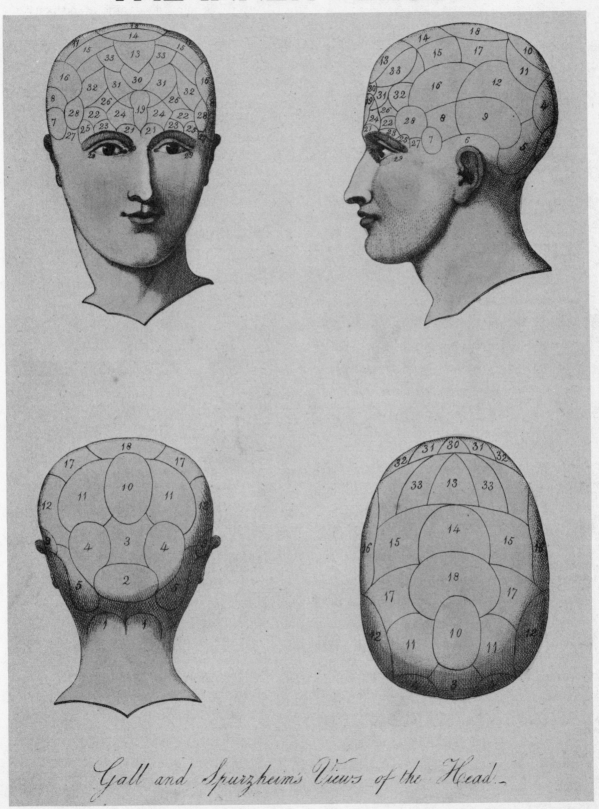

Gall and Spurzheim's Views of the Head.

Appetite Depressants

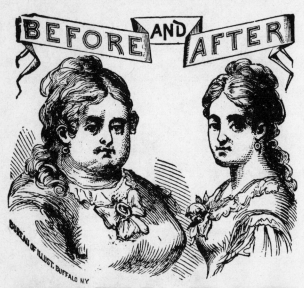

If you're living on a steady regimen of diet foods and supplements, you can get pretty hungry, and sometimes it seems like there's nothing you can do to make that empty feeling go away. So what about diet pills and other diet aids?

Walk into any drugstore and you'll see whole racks loaded with appetite depressants. I've never tried any of the over-the-counter diet pills, capsules, cookies, or gum, so here I can't speak from experience.

Here, very briefly, is a small listing of all diet foods and helpers on the market. The listings are by no means complete. I suggest you check your local supermarket and drug store to find out what they carry.

Use your good common sense when you shop, read the labels and if there are any questions talk to your doctor.

You must have common sense. I can tell. You bought this book.

THOMPSON MEDICAL COMPANY, INC.
919 Third Avenue
New York, New York 10022

Remember that there are no drug products—neither prescription drugs nor nonprescription (over-the-counter) drugs—that will *reduce* weight. You must cut down your dietary intake to lose weight. The following drug products are sold over the counter to help you decrease your dietary intake.

"APPEDRINE"   42 tablets $2.98

Contains: Phenylpropanolamine HCL 25 mg.
Caffeine 100 mg.
Sodium CarboxyMethylcellulose 50 mg.
Plus various vitamins

Directions: (Adults) One tablet thirty minutes before each meal with a full glass of water.

A diet plan and calorie-counter are enclosed.

"DEXATRIM"   56 capsules   (price unavailable)

A one-a-day timed-release capsule.
Contains: Phenylpropanolamine HCE 50 mg.
Caffeine 200 mg.

Directions: (Adults) Take one Dexatrim capsule at midmorning with a full glass of water.

A diet plan and calorie-counter are enclosed.

"VITA-SLIM"   50 capsules $5.95

Contains: Amphadrine (phenylpropanolamine HCL) 50 mg.
Also contains vitamins, iron, kelp, and lecithin.

Directions: (Adults) One capsule at 10 A.M. and one capsule at 4 P.M., each with a full glass of water.

A diet plan and calorie-counter are enclosed.

"PROLAMINE"   20 capsules $2.98

Contains: Phenylpropanolamine HCL 35 mg.
Caffine 140 mg.

Directions: Take one capsule at 10 A.M. and one capsule at 4 P.M. A diet plan and calorie-counter are enclosed.

"ANOREXIN"   50 capsules   (price unavailable)

Contains: Phenylpropanolamine HCL 25 mg.
Caffeine 100 mg.

Directions: (Adults) One capsule three times a day, one hour before each meal, with a full glass of water.

A diet plan and calorie-counter are enclosed.

"SLIM-LINE DIET PLAN CANDY"   36 pieces $1.98

Available in various flavors.

Ingredients: benzocaine, methylcellulose, corn syrup, sucrose, sweetened condensed skimmed milk, vegetable oil, mono- and di-glycerides, lecithin, salt, natural and artificial flavoring,

Analysis: available carbohydrates 82.1%, fat 7.3%, protein 1.5%. Each piece has approximately 21 calories.

Directions: You are to eat one or two pieces of candy with various beverages before meals, after meals, and between meals. A diet plan and calorie-counter are enclosed.

"SLIM-MINT FLAVORED CHEWING GUM"   36 Tablets   (price unavailable)

Active ingredients: benzocaine, essential oils, dextrose, methylcellulose.

Directions: Chew one or two pieces, then drink various beverages, before meals, after meals, and between meals. A diet plan and calorie-counter are enclosed.

The following explanations of some of the ingredients of the diet aids I have just discussed are supplied by the manufacturer, Thompson Medical Co., Inc.

Phenylpropanolamine HCL

Chemically similar to amphetamines but does not have the side effects. It inhibits appetite.

Methylcellulose

Is a noncaloric indigestible vegetable product that binds with water and gives a feeling of fullness.

Benzocaine

A topical anesthetic that anesthetizes the taste buds in the throat and mouth.

Caffeine

A stimulant and diuretic. One cup of coffee contains 100 mg. of caffeine.

If I were you, though, I'd stick to the natural stuff. Liquids are good fillers—whether the liquid is water, black coffee, tea, or diet soda pop; and my favorite low-calorie filler-uppers are sauerkraut, dill pickles and dill tomatoes, and cantaloupe. Pickles are especially good. They pop, crunch, drip on your shirt, and make your jaws work.

"As when a man dreams he is eating
And awakens with his hunger not satisfied,
Or as when a thirsty man dreams he is drinking
And awakes faint, with his thirst not quenched,
So shall the multitude of all nations be
That fight against Mount Zion."

Isaiah 29:8

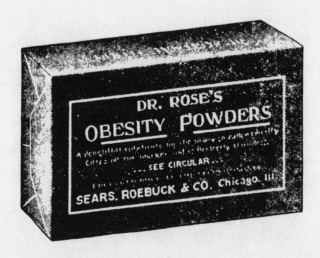

Diet Foods

Are You Fat?

Kellogg's Obesity Food Will Reduce Your Weight to Normal, Free You From Suffering and Turn Your Fat Into Muscle.

It Has Done This for Many Others Who Testify to its Efficacy — Trial Package Free.

Don't be fat. It is an abnormal and diseased condition of the body. Nutriment that should have built up bone and muscle for you has made fat instead.

Excess fat is attended by many dangers. The heart, stomach, liver, and kidneys become seri-

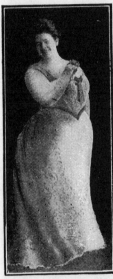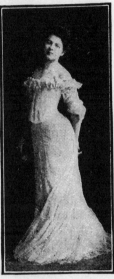

The Above Illustration Shows the Remarkable Effects of This Wonderful Obesity Food—What It Has Done for Others It Will Do for You.

ously affected; breathing is made difficult, and often, though seemingly well, the fat person is in grave danger.

Don't starve yourself. You will only become weakened and aggravate your condition without losing flesh.

There is a sure way and a safe way. Hundreds of reputable people testify to what Kellogg's Obesity Food has done for them. It has turned their fat into muscle. They submit their photographs as corroborative evidence. Can you doubt such proof?

Don't be fat. Write to me to-day and I will send you free, a trial package, postpaid, in plain wrapper.

One happy woman, Mrs. Mary Smith, 275 Sheldon St., Grand Rapids, Mich., says:

"My Dear Mr. Kellogg:

"I am sending you two of my photos. They will tell you better than I can how much different I look, and you can imagine how much better I feel.

"My doctor tells me that the effect of the remedy seems to be to strengthen and fortify the system before stripping it of its surplus fat. He was very much interested in the 'experiment,' as he called it. In fact, I do not believe I would have ordered it if he had not urged me to. He said that he had analyzed it and found it to be harmless, but that he didn't believe it could do what you claimed for it.

"I weighed over two hundred pounds, which, for a woman of my height, is very fat. Now I weigh 135, am plump and well formed, and I feel good all day long and sleep so restfully at night.

"I shall always thank you for what you have done for me, and I will be glad to have you refer me to any of your patients."

Right up here at the top of the page, I'm going to tell you that I'm not thrilled with the sweetening of saccharin. The aftertaste is not pleasant. I know it's the only non-nutritive sweetener we have left since the government took cyclamates off the market. (And it may be gone by the time you read this—see the note below.) What I don't understand is why, considering the profit potential of a new artificial sweetener, the pharmaceutical houses have not come up with anything yet. From what I've read there are many firms working on such a sweetener, but none is on the market. Let's get hot, gang, and help us out. (This has been an editorial.)

Many people I've talked to who have gotten used to diet foods and drinks say that the sugar-sweetened variety is distasteful to them now. The real stuff is too sweet. The same thing happened to me when I tried a glass of regular milk after having drunk skim milk for years. It tasted like a glass of heavy cream. Fortunately, I finally got used to diet soda pop. With the calories that I've saved, it was worth the struggle.

As you know, the diet food and drink business runs into hundreds of millions of dollars. There are hundreds of diet products out in almost every possible variety of food and drink, and they're a good way to save calories. Most supermarkets have a diet section on their shelves and in the frozen food cabinet. Give them a try.

Note: The Food and Drug Administration announced the ban of saccharin as this book was going to press. Whether or not that ban will be sustained remains an open question at this writing. The American public reacted with anguish and outrage at the prospect of having their saccharin products taken away, and questions were raised concerning the methodology and relevance of the study which led to the ban. Since the outcome is still unknown, no products were eliminated from this book because of their saccharin content. But do check the label of any dietetic product you might want to buy if you are concerned about saccharin.

METRECAL PRODUCTS

Metrecal was introduced in 1959—first as a liquid that was supposed to taste like a milkshake, then in "ice cream" form and in cookies. I was probably their first customer on earth. It was what I was waiting for—a measured dietetic meal that tasted fairly good. I ate so many of the cookies I think I o.d.'d on them. But there are only 230 calories in nine of them, so the guilt quotient was considerably lower than for regular cookies.

Metrecal has now expanded its line to include Metrecal Powders, Liquids, Wafers, Soups, Milk Shakes, Cookies, Diet Dinners, and Shape Liquid and Powder. You should be able to find them in most markets and drug stores.

NATURSLIM
Distributed by A & G Associates Inc.
136-45 37th Avenue
Flushing, New York 11354

NaturSlim is a powdered natural food supplement that is 86 percent protein, 2.5 percent carbohydrates, and 1.5 percent fat. Each two-tablespoon serving contains 70 calories, 17 grams of protein, 1 gram of carbohydrates, and no fat. It has no sugar either.

The NaturSlim program involves using the product for breakfast and lunch, mixed with low-fat milk or unsweetened juice, and eating a balanced meal for dinner. The NaturSlim people suggest you stay away from white bread and sugar.

They also include recipes for NaturSlim you can whip up in your blender. You can make such exotic concoctions as mocha shakes, yogurt shakes, and choco/maple shakes.

The thirty-day package consists of the NaturSlim food and a bottle of special formulated B–6 tablets. This provides forty to sixty meals, depending on how chubby you are. The cost is $19.95.

GET TRIM COMPANY
6515-A Corporate Drive
Houston, Texas 77036

Get Trim is a whole food in concentrated form that provides all the minimum daily requirements for adult health.

The program, which costs $19.95, consists of a one-month supply of Get Trim food, Vitamin B–6 and complete instructions. There is also a ten-day money-back guarantee.

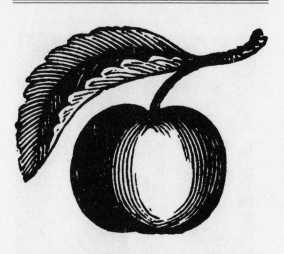

NUTRISLIM
221 Old Orchard Professional Building
Skokie, Illinois 60076

NutriSlim is a powder composed of soya, casein, and lactalbumin. It's 88 percent protein, 100 percent natural, and contains no drugs.

NutriSlim's weight-loss program consists of mixing the NutriSlim Powder with either eight ounces of 2-percent milk or six ounces of juice as a substitute for breakfast or lunch. For dinner you are to eat a balanced meal. You follow this for several days, and then the program is modified.

When you buy the NutriSlim Powder you also get B–6 vitamin pills. You are to take one of these with each meal.

A thirty-day supply of the powder and vitamins costs $18.60. A ten-day supply is $9.75. The company will also send you free literature if you're interested.

GET SLIM INTERNATIONAL, INC.
1415 Hurley
Fort Worth, Texas 76104

Get Slim International's weight-reducing plan basically is to eat one low-calorie meal a day, preferably dinner. The other two meals, breakfast and lunch, are to be fruit juice or low-fat milk along with Get Slim Powder.

Get Slim Powder is 86 percent protein and contains 74 calories per level tablespoon.

According to the label on Get Slim Powder, these are the ingredients; "A pure edible whole protein food of high biological value and low fat and carbohydrate content. A blended combination of Isolated Soy Protein, Calcium Caseinate, Sodium Caseinate, Lecithin, Magnesium Sulfate, Artificial & Natural Flavors, Kelp, Yeast, Lactalbumin, Niacin, Potassium Carbonate, Thiamine, Riboflavin, Pantothenic Acid, Choline, Pyridoxine, Biotin, Papain and Bromelain supplying a well balanced proportion of the Amino Acids and various B-Complex vitamins."

Also available are Get Slim Vitamin & Mineral Formula tablets that are to be taken with each meal—a total of three per day.

The price for the complete program is $16.00 ($9.00 for one pound of powder and $7.00 for the vitamin and mineral supplement) which will last approximately one month.

JOE WEIDER PRODUCTS
21100 Erwin Street
Woodland Hills, California 91364

Joe specializes in body-building and pumping iron, but he does have several low-calorie, weight-loss drinks:

Low-Calorie Breakfast Drink

This is the way body-builders can lose weight and still get proper nutrition. One ten-ounce can has 307 calories, 40 grams of carbohydrates, 30 grams of protein, and 3 grams of fat, plus vitamins and minerals. You can have vanilla or chocolate flavors. Twelve cans cost $12.98, sent freight collect.

Weight Loss XR7 Liquid

A slimmer's "meal in a can" that comes in chocolate, vanilla, and banana. Each ten-ounce can has 230 calories, 27 grams of carbohydrates, and 30 grams of protein, plus vitamins and minerals. Included is a fourteen-day reducing and shape-up course . . . showing you "how to muscle up while slimming down." A two-week supply is $12.98, sent freight collect. Weight Loss XR7 also comes in powder form too. One can makes four glasses when mixed with a quart of milk. One glass supplies 200 calories, 25 grams of carbohydrates, and 20 grams of protein. Comes in vanilla, chocolate, and strawberry. A fourteen-day supply costs $16.98, sent freight collect.

Whether you're a lifter or not, these could work for you. For myself, I'll just lift the can and develop a 10-inch waist.

Think about it: since the yield of a pound of fat is 3500 calories, an extra cookie each day for a year will make you 2½ pounds fatter next year than you were this year.

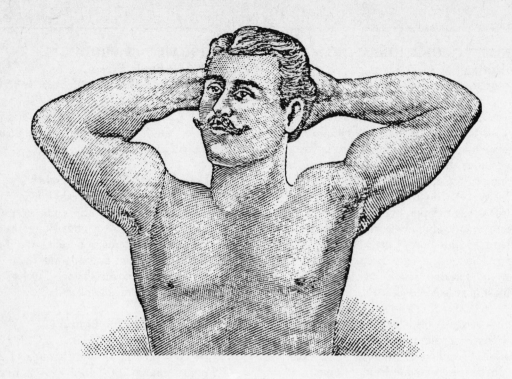

YORK HEALTH PRODUCTS, INC.
589 N.W. 62nd Street
Miami, Florida 33150

When I was growing up in Kansas City, almost every guy I knew was "working out with weights" in the basement. Not having that much energy and knowing that all that work would make me even hungrier, I would sit in a chair on the side with a bag of Hydrox cookies and a quart of chocolate milk and kibbitz. I wish some of my friends had gone in for York Health Products equipment, because in addition to the standard barbells, weights, exercise boards and such groan makers as the York Adjustable Krusher Grip, Heavy Duty Tricep Bar Exerciser, Iron Health Shoes, complete home gyms, and a little number called "Arm Blasters," they also carry a line of Bob Hoffman's Food Supplements. We dieters are concerned with only two:

Hoffman's Hi-Proteen Reducing Plan
Formula
This comes in either one-pound containers of powder or tablet form. You can have either in vanilla or chocolate. Mix eight ounces with a quart of water and drink throughout the day instead of eating three meals. Total calories: 840. Or you can eat one meal and substitute the Reducing Formula for the other two

meals. The powder costs $2.35 for one pound. The cost of 400 tablets is $3.00; 900 tablets, $5.75.

Hoffman's Super Hi-Proteen Diet Bar
Comes plain or chocolate-covered, and the cost for a box of eight is $2.40. The ingredients and vitamins in these bars run as long as your arm. This is a candy-like product with such goodies as honey, peanut butter, soy flour, and skim milk powder. I'd like to give you some more of the ingredients, but I'm writing this late at night and I'm starting to twitch from hunger.

York also includes with each box of their candy bars a three-page brochure on fructose, a pure sugar which occurs naturally in many fruits and which is much sweeter than sucrose or glucose sweeteners—therefore you use less. Fructose helps relieve the dieting symptoms of hunger: stress, headaches, and weakness. And, if you take it in small amounts frequently throughout the day while you eat very small portions of meats, salads, and fats (supplemented by vitamins), it will help burn the carbohydrates more quickly. So, if fructose is taken as directed, according to the York brochure, "a substantial weight loss should result within a few days without the stress associated with other diets."

TASTI DIET FOOD PRODUCTS
At your local supermarket

Tasti Diet has almost a complete supermarket of diet foods for you to choose from. There are approximately fifty Tasti Diet food products ranging from chocolate topping, pancake mix, and mayonnaise to diced carrots, salad dressings, Concord grape jelly, and sliced peaches. They even have "Eggstra," a fresh-egg substitute which has 75 percent less cholesterol, 75 percent less fat, and 45 percent fewer calories than fresh eggs.

Tasti Diet products have no sugar added to them. They also control the carbohydrate and calorie levels during the packing process.

The next time you're in your supermarket, stroll over to the diet-food section and check it out. I'm sure you'll find enough Tasti Diet products to make your own low calorie banquet.

COOKING EASE
At your local supermarket

Cooking Ease is a natural vegetable cooking spray that can be used just like oil, butter, margarine, or shortening in all kinds of cooking to keep foods from sticking.

Plus Cooking Ease has only ten calories per two- to three-second spray. Compare that to one tablespoon of butter, with 100 calories, or cooking oil, with 125 calories. It can make fried foods taste and look like fried foods without loads of calories or that greasy taste.

Get a can and spray yourself thin. I sprayed some in my hair figuring its natural butter aroma might attract some nice plump ladies.

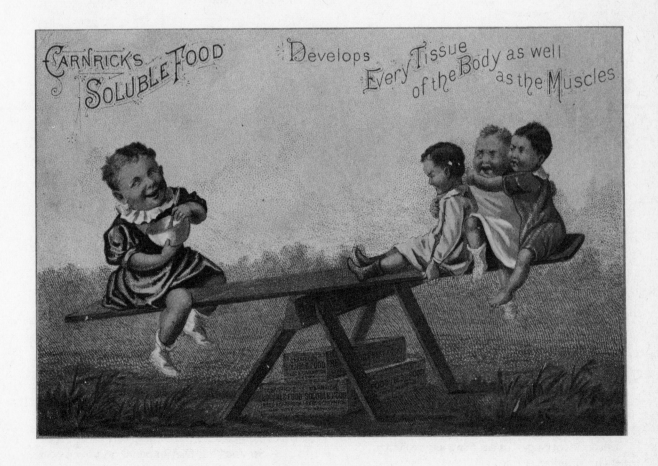

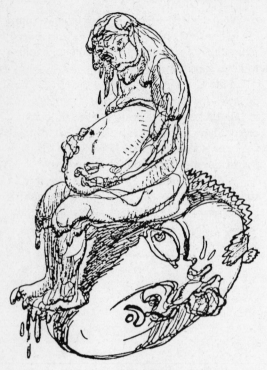

Man, Made of Butter
Buttermensch

Sweet 'N Low puts out a whole slew of goodies for you: a little vinyl case to carry your packets in your pocket or purse; "Cooking with Sweet 'N Low Recipe Booklet"; Sweet 'N Low "Togetherness" recipe book featuring cookies, cakes and frosting; "Sweet 'N Low Holiday Recipes"; "7 Festive Ways to Save Calories"; "34 Ways to Cheat on Your Sugar with Sweet 'N Low Home Canning and Freezing Recipes"; "New Sweet 'N Low Brown Granulated Sugar Recipe Sampler"; and a "Sweet 'N Low Calorie Counter." Now that's a real smorgasbord of free goods.

SUCARYL ARTIFICIAL SWEETENER
Abbott Laboratories
Abbott Park
North Chicago, Illinois 60064

Sucaryl is a sodium-saccharin-based artificial sweetener. It's sold in both liquid and tablet forms. The suggested retail prices are:

6 oz.	$1.49
12 oz.	2.29
20 oz.	3.29
100 ct.	.96
200 ct.	1.69
1,000 ct.	4.33

You can also request a free recipe booklet for liquid Sucaryl from Abbott Laboratories, D-792, at the address above.

SWEET 'N LOW
Cumberland Packing Corporation
2 Cumberland Street
Brooklyn, New York 11205

The package says: "New Sweet 'N Low—no bitter after-taste sugar substitute—a blend of nutritive and non-nutritive sweeteners—Use one packet of Sweet 'N Low for the sweetness of two teaspoons of sugar in hot and cold drinks, fruits, cereals and cooking. Each packet contains approximately 9/10 gram of carbohydrates equivalent to about 3½ calories. This should be taken into account by diabetics.

"Ingredients: Nutritive lactose, 4% soluble saccharin—a non-nutritive artificial sweetener which should be used only by persons who must restrict their intake of ordinary sweets (40 milligrams per packet or 20 milligrams per each teaspoon of sugar sweetening equivalency), cream of tartar.

"Approximate Analysis: No protein. No fat. Available carbohydrates 94%."

DIET IMPERIAL MARGARINE
Lever Brothers
390 Park Avenue
New York, New York 10022

One tablespoon of Diet Imperial Margarine has 45 calories and no cholesterol, and it's made of 34 percent vegetable oil.

For comparison with regular margarine, I whipped out my handy calorie-counter and discovered that some regular margarines have over 100 calories per tablespoon.

So slap that Diet Imperial on your bagel, and hold the cream cheese.

SUGARLO COMPANY
3540 Atlantic Avenue
P.O. Box 1017
Atlantic City, New Jersey 08404

SugarLo has the products that will give that sweet tooth a good workout and not expand the tummy department. They manufacture SugarLo Diet Fruit Yogurts, SugarLo Ice Milk, SugarLo Ice Cream, and SugarLo artificial sweetener packets.

SugarLo Diet Fruit Yogurts

These have only 50 percent of the calories of other fruit yogurts. They have no sucrose or dextrose, and average only 6 percent carbohydrates, all of it as natural milk sugar and natural fruit sugar. Additional sweetening is supplied by saccharin. You may spoon up raspberry, strawberry, pineapple, black cherry, or blueberry.

SugarLo Ice Milk

Contains no added sugar. One hundred grams of SugarLo Dietetic Ice Milk contains 120 calories, as opposed to 261 calories for ice cream that contains 18 percent fat. How about a dishful of vanilla, coffee, chocolate, lemon chiffon, or raspberry?

SugarLo Ice Cream

Also contains no added sugar and has 180 calories per 100 grams. Regular ice cream has 261 calories. SugarLo Ice Cream comes in chocolate, vanilla, coffee, lemon chiffon, strawberry, and orange-pineapple.

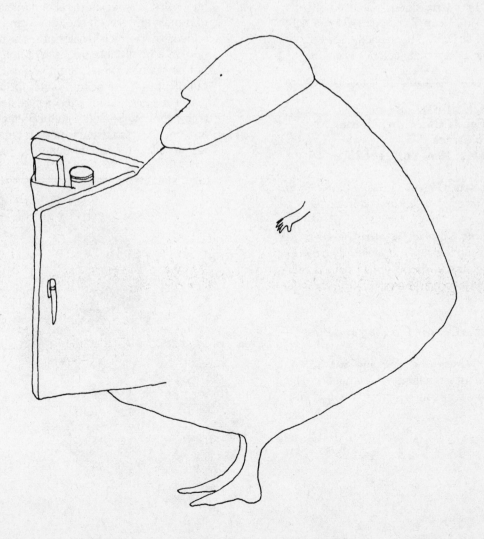

THINNY-THIN DIETARY FROZEN DESSERT
Sold at Carvel Ice Cream Stores

A low-calorie frozen dessert that has only 18.5 calories per fluid ounce. It's 99 percent fat-free, low in carbohydrates, and made with fresh dairy ingredients, and contains no artificial sweeteners. Flavors are vanilla, chocolate, mint, strawberry, and coffee.

SHIMMER GELATIN DESSERT
Louis Sherry, Inc.
18 West Putnam Avenue
Greenwich, Connecticut 06830

"Stay Slimmer with Shimmer" is a free booklet of fourteen recipes from Louis Sherry, Inc., using different flavors of Shimmer low-calorie gelatin.

You'll quiver with delight at the Pink Cloud Dessert: Prepare 1 package Shimmer, raspberry or cherry flavor. Chill till slightly thickened. Add 1 cup plain yogurt. Beat till light and fluffy. Pile lightly into serving dishes. Eight half-cup servings, twenty calories each.

NUTRITION SERVICES
General Foods Consumer Center
250 North Street
White Plains, New York 10625

All right, dieters, General Foods has three food products that are labeled low-calorie:

D-Zerta Low Calorie Gelatin Dessert
Half a cup has eight calories and no carbohydrates. You can spoon up six different flavors; strawberry, raspberry, cherry, orange, lemon, and lime.

D-Zerta Low Calorie Pudding and Pie Filling
Better check the package for calorie counts and other nutrition information. This dessert comes in vanilla, chocolate, and butterscotch.

D-Zerta Low Calorie Whipped Topping Mix
One tablespoon has eight calories and no carbohydrates. Spray it on lots of low-calorie desserts.

For you rabbit-food mavens who like crunchy salads, there is Good Seasons Low Calorie Italian Salad Dressing Mix. One tablespoon has eight calories and two grams of carbohydrate.

PETER PAN LOW-SODIUM PEANUT BUTTER
Swift & Company
1919 Swift Drive
Oak Brook, Illinois 60521

Peanut butter has always been one of my all-time favorite goodies. Whip out the p.b., a jar of grape jelly, and a loaf of soft white bread—I could be dancing into nirvana.

Now Peter Pan has a low-sodium peanut butter that is an economical and quality source of protein and has no cholesterol and no sugar added. There are 140 calories in one serving of one and a half tablespoons. You may or may not be saving calories, but if you're on a low-salt diet this is the peanut butter for you.

You can send for a recipe booklet giving a recipe for Low Sodium Peanut Butter Cookies, and you can also use this peanut butter in any recipe calling for peanut butter.

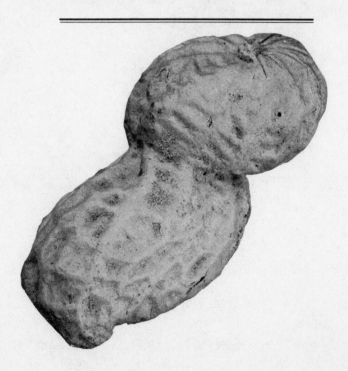

ALBA PRODUCTS
Alba Foods Company, Inc.
880 Third Avenue
New York, New York 10022

Alba has a number of low-calorie products available:

Alba Instant Nonfat Dry Milk

Pure cow's milk, with only the fat and water removed. It is fortified with Vitamins A and D in accordance with government regulations. Eight fluid ounces contain 80 calories.

Chocolate Alba Instant Nonfat Dry Milk

Sugar-free chocolate drink. Again, 80 calories in eight fluid ounces.

Alba '77 Fit 'N Frosty

Sugar-free, comes in chocolate, vanilla and strawberry. Seventy calories in twelve fluid ounces.

Alba '66 Hot Cocoa Mix

Sugar-free. Seventy calories in six fluid ounces.

Alba has about forty-five low-calorie recipes based on Alba products (what else?). Some of these recipes sound scrumptious: Chilled Cucumber Soup (very elegant), Chocolate Malt (use chocolate diet soda pop, sugar substi-

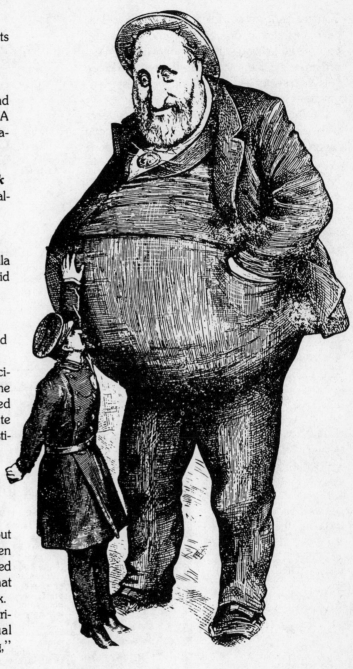

tute, Alba milk, and ice cubes; beat the hell out of it in a blender—um-um), Baked Chicken Florentine (just like the old country), Baked Custard (usual, but yummy). Amazing what you can do with those little packets of dry milk.

Alba also publishes little "Tips on Nutrition" flyers such as "Sugar Can Equal Danger," "Adding New Life to Milk Drinking," and "Sugar's Costly Calories."

ESTEE CANDY CO., INC.
169 Lackawanna Avenue
Parsippany, New Jersey 07054

Tongue hanging out for a delicious chocolate bar? Just dying for one little chocolate chip cookie? I'll tell you what I'm going to do. We'll scream for Estee to come to the rescue. Estee bills themselves as "The World's Largest Manufacturer of Dietetic Sweets."

What does Estee sweeten their sweets with? I quote from their letter: "Estee Dietetic Sweets are made without sugar, salt, corn syrup or artificial sweeteners of any kind. In their place, we use mannitol and sorbitol—the natural sweet, nutritive ingredients found in many fruits and edible berries." They also add, "This information is set forth for the medical profession; consumers should always consult their physicians as to its use in their diets."

Estee offers a variety of goodies: Dietetic Gum Drops, Dietetic Hard Candies, Dietetic Chocolate Bars, Dietetic Candy Coated Chocolate, Dietetic Boxed Chocolates, Sugarless Mints, Sugarless Gum, Sugarless Bubble Gum (oh, boy), and Dietetic Cookies and Wafers. Some sample calorie counts: Estee Sour Lemon Sugarless Hard Candy has 12 calories per piece, an Estee Dietetic Milk Chocolate Flavored Wafer has 110, Estee Sugarless Peppermint Gum has 7 per stick, and Estee Dietetic Chocolate Chip Cookies have 30 calories each. They taste pretty good and they save you lots of evil calories. If you can't find them in your local stores, write Estee and they'll send you everything you need to order their products by mail.

THE COSMOPOLITAN.

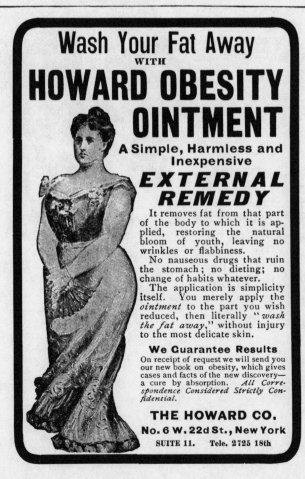

SHASTA BEVERAGES
26901 Industrial Boulevard
Hayward, California 94545

The Diet Shasta Recipe Book, "A Well-Rounded Collection of Slimming Recipes" (that's my kind of joke) is a bunch of diet recipes from Diet Shasta Soda Pop. One of the thirteen different flavors of Diet Shasta is used in each recipe.

Many of the diet recipes come from readers across the country. The Diet Shasta Test Kitchens have provided the rest.

What fascinated me about this booklet is that there are recipes for salads, soups, vegetables, entrées, desserts, spreads, and toppings. I always thought that the only foods you could make with diet soda would be desserts. There's a lot of creativity in what Shasta's done.

Let me give you some samples: Mocha Polka (made with Diet Shasta Creme Soda, dry milk, instant coffee, and a little salt); Chicken Salad à la Tarragon (made with chicken and vegetables and topped with Creamy Tarragon Dressing, the dressing has as one of its ingredients Diet Shasta Ginger Ale); Beef Stuffed Zucchini (made with Diet Shasta Ginger Ale), and Pineapple "Cheesecake" (prepared with Diet Shasta Lemon-Lime).

SOUTHEND
suits me alright
already getting STOUT AND BETTER

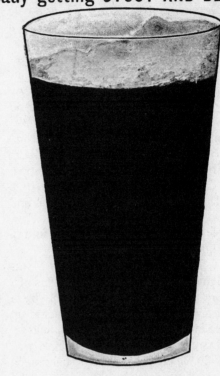

According to some recent research by Dr. Jules Hirsch of Rockefeller University in New York, overfeeding a child early in life appears to increase the number and size of fat cells in his body. This enlarged population of fat cells is not reduced by dieting later in life; only the size of the cells diminishes with weight loss. An extremely fat person, says Hirsch, may have five times the normal number of fat cells. Even when these cells shrink during weight loss, they seem to remain "hungry" and ready to be filled up again, which may partly explain why some fat people cannot keep off the pounds they shed.

NO-CAL CORPORATION
112-02 15th Avenue
College Point, New York 11356

You're struggling up a huge sand dune on the Sahara Desert, your mouth is as dry as a bale of cotton, and every pore is screaming for a long cool drink of soda pop—but you're overweight and you can't have any of those sugar-filled goodies. But there, before your sunburned eyes, glimmers a No-Cal oasis serving seventeen different flavors of dietetic soda. And each flavor has less than one calorie per bottle. Your parched lips can choose from Cola, Ginger, Black Cherry, Black Raspberry, Chocolate, Chocolate Mint, Root Beer, Orange, Grape, Cream, Coffee, Club Soda, Tonic Water, Citrus, Pink Grapefruit, Red Pop, and Shape-Up (lemon with a hint of lime). Plus, they're all approved by leading weight-control groups and diabetic associations.

No-Cal was started in 1952 when Morris Kirsch, a member of the board of directors of a New York hospital, was approached by a group of doctors who asked him to come up with a "palatable sugar-free soft drink." His father, Hyman, started out in the soft-drink business in 1904, when he delivered his handmade flavored soft drinks by horse and wagon, so the doctors must have figured that Morris would know everything worth knowing about soft drinks.

The "Savers Cookbook," published by No-Cal, is a thirty-two-page low-calorie cookbook that shows you how to save calories at breakfast, lunch, dinner, and the cocktail hour. Wake up to a strawberry omelet using No-Cal Strawberry Butter (which you've made with No-Cal Strawberry soda) at only 170 calories per serving.

At lunch you can dine on a Jubilee Salad made with apples, celery, any flavor of No-Cal except Cherry or Coffee, unflavored gelatin, cold water, and boiling water—22 calories per serving.

If you're an elbow-bender, your parched lips can be refreshed by a No-Cal Creole Cooler, No-Cal Party Punch, or a No-Cal Temperance Daisy.

At dinner you can have Western Barbecued Chicken, made with No-Cal Black Cherry (290 calories per portion), or Baked Fish Fillets with Apples, made with one pack of No-Cal Granulated Sweetener (232 calories per serving), or many other main dishes enhanced by No-Cal sodas.

A little something sweet afterwards? Try the Cheese Blintzes with Cherry Sauce. Only 200 calories per serving. . . . Regular blintzes with cherry sauce have 350 calories. You can pull your Gucci belt in a notch after that whopping 150-calorie saving.

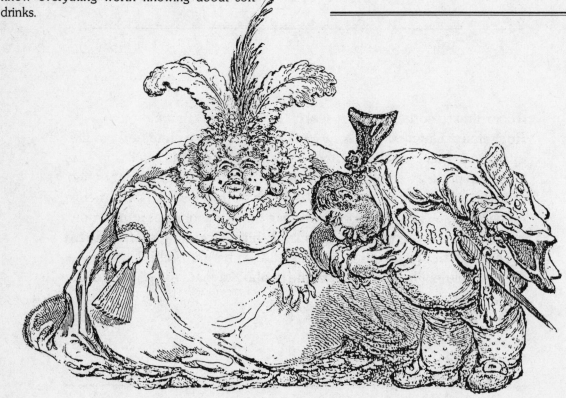

WEIGHT WATCHERS PRODUCTS
At your local supermarket

Weight Watchers Apple Snack

This is the only snack approved by Weight Watchers. I guess it's supposed to keep you away from potato chips and pretzels. Apple Snacks are bite-size pieces of dehydrated apple that are made without removing its natural flavor. Each package contains the equivalent of one medium-size apple. That means you're only eating about fifty calories.

Weight Watchers Fruit Snack

These are also made from dehydrated apples, but they are given different flavors, so that you can choose from strawberry, peach, and cinnamon. You can pick up a package and skip down the street munching all the way.

Weight Watchers Thin Sliced Bread

There is nothing low-calorie about the content of this bread, but you still save calories because two slices of Weight Watchers Bread equal one slice of regular sliced bread. It's sliced extra thin, you see. You might be able to get a little recipe book on different ways to use this bread. It's called "12 Great Ways to Enjoy Weight Watchers Thin Sliced Enriched Bread."

Weight Watchers Soft Drinks

You can gurgle down thirteen different flavors: lemon-lime, cherry cola, grape, root beer, black cherry, creme, chocolate, cola, raspberry creme, ginger ale, strawberry, orange, and Frosta, whatever, that is. There is no fat, protein, vitamins, or minerals in any of the flavors. Each flavor contains from 8.2 to 9.1 miligrams per fluid ounce of sodium saccharin as a sweetener.

Weight Watchers Frozen Dessert

This Frozen Dessert has 20 calories per fluid ounce and no artificial sweeteners. It is also almost cholesterol-free, containing less than one percent fat. One portion counts as four fluid ounces of skim milk and one fruit on the Weight Watchers Program (see page 129). I haven't tried it yet, but it's supposed to taste like ice cream. You can choose from vanilla, chocolate, or Neopolitan; the dessert comes packed in half gallons or Snack Cups. Write to Public Relations, Camargo Foods, Inc., 5020 Spring Grove Avenue, Cincinnati, Ohio 45232 for "Frozen Dessert Recipes."

Other Weight Watchers Products

Cheese and Prima Pizza (frozen), Skim Milk, Lowfat Cottage Cheese, Extracts, Sauces, Gravies, Seasonings, and Salad Dressing Mixes.

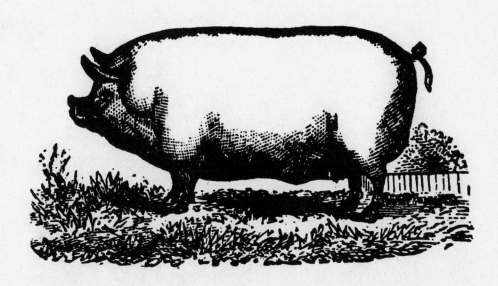

ROY CLARK'S DIETER'S CHOICE
Low-calorie and low-carbohydrate foods

Anyone who has watched much television in the last five years knows that Roy Clark is a formerly chunky country-and-western singer who has had a weight-control problem all his life. Good ole boy Roy has now come out with a whole mess of low-calorie and low-carbohydrate packaged dinners, plus a catsup and three salad dressings.

The initial five frozen dinners are: cooked veal stew (calories, 195; carbohydrates, 2.31 grams); chili without beans (calories, 120; carbohydrates, 2.35 grams); breast of chicken in barbecue sauce (calories, 157.5; carbohydrates, 2.10 grams); chicken chow mein without noodles (calories, 195; carbohydrates, 3.89 grams); and poached fillet of fish with spinach (calories, 202.5; carbohydrates, 2.98 grams). More varieties are scheduled for the future.

The French, garlic, and Italian dressings offer 1.5 calories per ounce; the imitation catsup, 2.5 calories.

So tune up your fat banjo, pardner, and have a good feed.

Diet Restaurants and Diet Food Stores

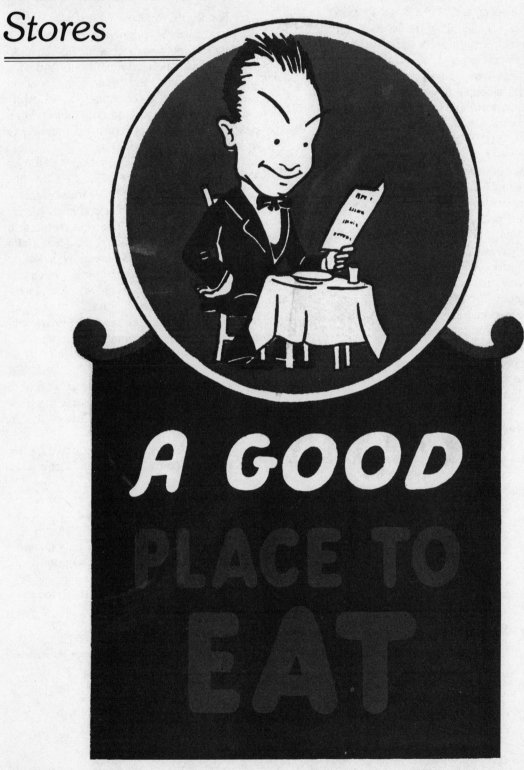

A GOOD PLACE TO EAT

I've been able to find very few diet restaurants—that is, restaurants devoted to serving diet foods exclusively. But many restaurants have a few diet items on their regular menu. For instance, in my pizzerias I serve a Diet Riot. This consists of the top of a mushroom, onion, and green pepper pizza with tomatoes and three ounces of cheese. It's like a stew baked in a pan. Plus you get a large green salad with fresh lemon dressing and all the diet soda pop you can drink. The diet pizza has no dough or crust. The total calorie-count is approximately 400, and after you eat it, you're stuffed. I invented it myself seven years ago and finally put it on the menu a couple of years ago.

The reason there aren't more diet restaurants is that when people go out to eat, they don't want to diet. This is another Goldberg Theory. But there are many serious dieters who must eat out with people who are not on diets. There should be something for them.

If you know of any diet restaurants or regular restaurants with unusual diet foods on the menu, please write and let me know.

Like diet restaurants, diet stores—that is, stores selling strictly diet-food products—are few and far between. I think there is a tremendous opportunity for someone to open diet stores. There are enough diet-food products now that an enterprising entrepreneur could open a small supermarket devoted exclusively to selling diet products. With the interest in dieting, someone could help overweight people and make a bundle.

Until that happens, supermarkets and health food stores are still your best sources of low-calorie foods. But be careful buying diet foods in health food stores. They carry a lot of high-calorie foods like nuts and dried fruits. Make sure that what you're buying is really low-calorie or dietetic.

THE DIET GOURMET SHOPPES OF AMERICA, INC.
121 East 57th Street, New York City
167 Lincoln Ave., Elberon, New Jersey
4770 Okeechobee Blvd., West Palm Beach, Florida
315 Millburn Ave., Millburn, New Jersey

Len Torine, the owner of the Diet Gourmet Shoppes, says he opened a diet restaurant because his wife, Susan, couldn't find anyplace dietetic to eat when they went out. And when she was pregnant with their son, Jonathan, Susan went up to 190 pounds. Then Len, the devoted slim husband, started making these delicious gourmet diet foods. So naturally he opened a diet restaurant.

The newest Diet Gourmet opened in New York City in the spring of 1977. It's a beautiful cafeteria restaurant with small round seats so you can tell when your rear end is shrinking.

They have a huge menu featuring such yummy numbers as a King Crab Meat Platter (240 calories), which is served with lettuce, tomato, cottage cheese, fruit, and crackers.

Or you can munch on an "Our Hero" sandwich (253 calories). Our Hero is made with pita bread, ham, cheese, and turkey with wine vinegar, lettuce, tomato, and spices.

For dessert there's Diet Gourmet's Low Fat Ice Cream, which they say is half the calories of regular ice cream. A regular cup is 65 calories and you can lick such exotic flavors as Milky Weigh, Peanut Butter Cup, and Very Strawberry.

They also have soups, Dannon Low Fat Soft Frozen Yogurt, lots of sandwiches, and vegetable salads.

If you're one of the kids on one of the diet group diets, they'll even weigh everything for you.

I tried the Peanut Butter Cup ice cream. And let me tell you that it was so good I saw stars.

Besides, Mr. Torine says that 70 percent of his customers are women. I plan to hang around there a lot.

SKINNY GOURMET—DIET FOODS AND DESSERTS

In California: San Francisco, San Mateo, Santa Clara, San Jose, Fresno, Castro Valley, Monterey, San Rafael, and Santa Rosa.

In Arizona: Phoenix and Gendale

Suppose you could go into a restaurant and order barbecued chicken, salad, carrots or squash, a green vegetable, and a banana split—for total calories of approximately 700? You can: these plus many more low-calorie foods such as salads, Mexican food, fish, chicken, beef, and desserts are available at the Skinny Gourmet Restaurants.

These restaurants serve exclusively low-calorie foods. Just look at some of the goodies you can have with no guilt: Chili Con Carne (344 calories); Veal Cabbage Rolls (340 calories); Stuffed Chicken Breasts (470 calories); and Spaghetti and Meatballs (300 calories). And hold on to your sweet tooth. Skinny Gourmet offers fourteen different desserts, from a Hot Fudge Sundae (120 calories) to Peach Melba (159 calories).

The Skinny Gourmet has the blessing of Weight Watchers, TOPS, Diet Workshop, and the American Diabetes Association. They cater not just to low-calorie diets, but to low-sugar, low-sodium, or low-cholesterol diets, too.

Right now the Skinny Gourmet is only in the West, but they're planning to come east soon. Till then, California, here I come!

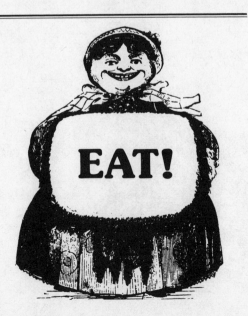

RICE'S DELI & LEGAL DIET EMPORIUM
4610 W. Burleigh Street
Milwaukee, Wisconsin 53210

Rice's Deli & Legal Diet Emporium (their motto: "Be a Rice Guy") is—oh my—like the federal government—divided into three parts.

1. Rice's Deli, which serves all sorts of fattening, wonderful foods.
2. Rice's Legal Diet Emporium: Beverly Rice, who along with her husband, Bruce, owns Rice's, lost 110 pounds with Weight Watchers several years ago. But then she had trouble finding permissible Weight Watchers foods when she went out to eat. Being in the delicatessen business already, Beverly and Bruce decided to add a "legal" Weight Watchers menu to their regular fattening menu. The diet menu has twenty legal goodies for you to choose from. Here's a couple of samples: Diet Chopped Liver (sandwich)—chopped liver, toast, and pickle for $1.75; and Vealburger on a Bun, with sliced raw onion, lettuce, and pickle for $1.75. There's something for every fatty, plus twenty legal side orders including diet potato salad and diet malts.

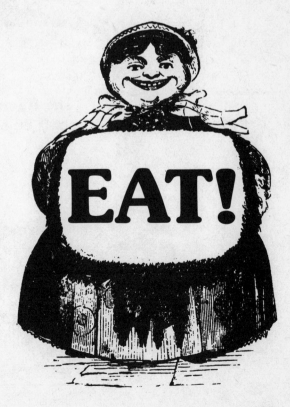

107

3. RICE'S LEGAL DIET COOK BOOK
P.O. Box 18422
Milwaukee, Wisconsin 53218
$3.95 Paperback 56 pages

Now I want you to pay close attention to what I'm going to tell you. The *Rice's Legal Diet Cook Book* contains over 240 recipes. Most of the recipes call for Rice's Legal Extracts or Rice's Legal Artificial Sweetner. The flavors are: almond, banana, black cherry, black walnut, blueberry, bourbon, brandy, butter, butter pecan, butter rum, butterscotch, cherry, chocolate, chocolate-mint, cinnamon, coconut, creme de menthe, gin, lemon, maple, maraschino cherry, mocha, peach, peanut butter, pistachio, pineapple, plum, raspberry, root beer, rum, scotch, sherry, strawberry, toffee, and (these are new flavors) anise, lime, orange, and wintergreen.

Here's a sample recipe from the book:

Strawberry Malt

½ cup whole strawberries
⅓ cup powdered milk
¼ cup cold water
1 teaspoon Rice's Legal Strawberry Extract
1 teaspoon Rice's Legal Raspberry Extract
1 teaspoon Rice's Legal Artificial Sweetner
1 drop red food coloring
1 or 1½ cups crushed ice

Blend all ingredients except ice at high speed until smooth. Add ice and blend again until smooth.

The extracts are $1 a bottle. The artificial sweetener is $1.29 a bottle. Minimum order is $6; add $1 for handling and delivery. Both extracts and sweetener can be ordered along with the cookbook from the address above.

To me, the whole idea of Rice's Diet Emporium, cookbook, extracts, and everything else is real "Rice."

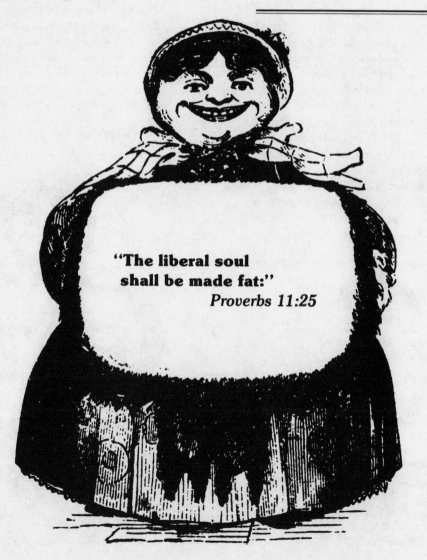

"The liberal soul shall be made fat:"
Proverbs 11:25

THIN'S INN
24-07 Broadway
Fairlawn, New Jersey

THIN'S INN
223 Route 18
E. Brunswick, New Jersey

All these stores are part of one company, and all of them have what you've been looking for—a big selection of about 200 low-calorie foods, including many of those favorite foods you never thought could be made with fewer calories. Let me get your juices flowing with some of the low-calorie goodies these stores offer:

Apple Strudel, sugar-free, 80 calories
Baked Ziti, sugar-free, 225 calories
Shrimp Chow Mein, sugar-free, 160 calories
Dietary Frozen Dessert—comes in 29 flavors—
    half the calories of regular ice cream, 99.5
    percent fat-free

THIN IS INN
177 Columbia Turnpike
Florham Park, New Jersey

DIET BAZAAR
1493 Weaver Street
Scarsdale, New York

Breakfast Veal Sausage, sugar-free, 40 calories
    for each one-ounce link

Although all these stores are in the East, many diet foods can be sold by mail, so write one of the stores for a list of their diet products if you can't shop in person. For each food on their lists, they offer a per portion breakdown of the sugar content, calories, carbohydrates, fats, and sodium so that you know exactly what you're getting and how the foods might fit into whatever diet plan you are following. In addition, some specialized information of interest to members of various weight-loss clubs is given.

LEAN LINE DIET DEN
1601 Park Avenue
South Plainfield, New Jersey 07080

Lean Line diet groups have come up with their own diet store called—what else—Lean Line Diet Den.

Lean Line doesn't want you to suffer even a little bit while your skinny pals are eating all those tasty ethnic and treat foods. They feel that misery doesn't have to be part of a successful diet. So they have devoted a whole store to such diet foods as the following.

Salads: Tuna, lobster, shrimp, chicken, cole slaw, and mock potato salad. (I never heard of a phony potato. I'm going to have to check that out.) Anyway, all the salads are made according to the Lean Line diet program.

Italian Lunches: Eggplant parmigiana, baked ziti, manicotti, stuffed shells, and lasagna.
Ice Cream: This is a frozen dietary dessert that comes in sixteen flavors; bulk-packed, plus cones and in sandwiches.
Slim Shake: Chocolate-malted-type drink with the same caloric value as an eight-ounce glass of skim milk.
Other foods: All-veal sausage, chow mein, delicatessen meats, cheesecakes and noncaloric desserts.

And all the gang that mans the store is well versed in the Lean Line Program and other diet programs, too.

THIN WEIGH DIET STORES
4025 S.W. 96th Avenue
Miami, Florida
Phone: (305) 223-7964

6738 Pembroke Road
Pembroke Pines, Florida
Phone: (305) 966-1899

Ah, to be in Miami. Sun, surf, bikinis, and two Thin Weigh stores to keep you tucked into those bikinis. The stores are diet grocery stores owned by a husband and wife combo.

Their sugar-free offerings include cheesecake, blintzes, pies, sundaes, and salad dressings. Thin Weigh stores also carry a complete line of calorie-controlled lunches, dinners, and seasonings, and a low-fat soft ice cream (made with a skim milk base). You can dine on such delicacies as Veal Balls Spaghetti (395 calories); Shrimp Chow Mein (255 calories); and Apple Pie (129 calories).

Everything in these stores is for weight reduction and all items are wrapped in individual portions, so there's no weighing or measuring. You can taste every product before buying, plus you get a money-back guarantee.

And the stores mail-order both dry items and frozen food all over the country. Write or phone for a list of what's available through the mail.

THREE
TECHNOLOGY

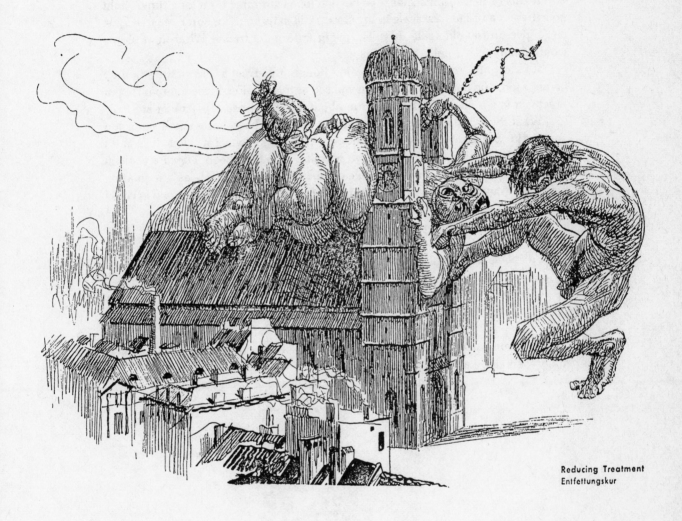

Reducing Treatment
Entfettungskur

Everyone, especially dieters, likes little machines, gadgets and gimmicks. Buying a diet gadget or machine doesn't guarantee you'll lose weight—you still have to cut down—but it can sure help by giving you something to mess around with until you're ready to eat. Keep those hands busy, busy, busy.

In my opinion a blender is an excellent tool for dieters. There are many delicious foods and drinks that can be whipped up in a blender. And they're fun to watch. Also, if you have to weigh what you eat, a good food scale can come in handy. As for bathroom scales, I've been in love with mine for a long time. Right now there is a brand-new scale in my closet, still in its box. For some reason, I just can't give up my old scale. It's like giving up a good friend. What kind of guy would dump an old pal?

If I was going to do it all over again, though, I'd invest in one of the stand-up balance jobs the doctors use. As you will see in this section, scale companies put these out in smaller models. They run about $100 in most department stores.

What the world needs now—and doesn't already have—is a small scale you can put in your suitcase and take with you. When I go away for a few days and I get up in the morning and can't weigh myself, I go a little bozo. I *need* a scale in the morning. I did *see* a portable scale once. It was the same size as a regulation bathroom scale but it had a canvas carrying bag. I'm sure the scale-makers could manufacture one much smaller.

Two other Goldberg Inventions that haven't been patented yet:

1. A diet belt with a calorie-counter on the inside and notches on the outside to tell you how you're doing.
2. A dieter's knife, fork and spoon set that swivels so the food won't stay on it and the food flops back on the plate.

If you can get either of these items off the drawing board, I'll buy one in a minute. Likewise a lightweight portable scale.

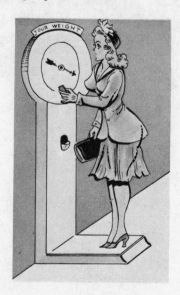

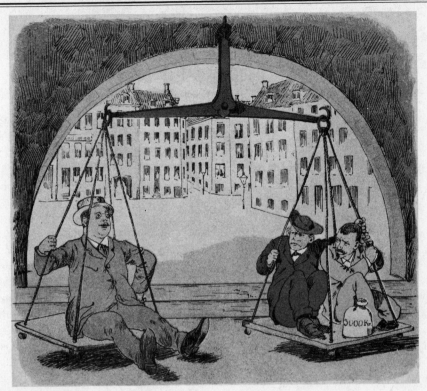

The Land of Ounce or Oz.

Once upon a time in the little village of Ounce, which was located forty-three miles southeast of Terre Haute, Indiana, there lived a family called the Harry Toledos. Now the Toledos were the richest folks in Oz. because they had The Magic Scale.

Chubby pilgrims journeyed from far and wide to be weighed on The Magic Scale. You may query, what was so magical about this scale? The secret of The Scale was that no matter what you ate, when you got on The Magic Scale, you still remained your ideal weight.

Around the Toledo cottage, Harry opened all sorts of food stands. You could eat juicy cheeseburgers, hot drippy pizza, crisp French fries, two-pound banana splits, warm Dutch apple pie, and rich dark brownies loaded with nuts. But regardless of how much you ate, you remained trim and svelte.

Sidney Greenstreet gave Harry Toledo The Magic Scale just before he went to the Big Diet Meeting in the Sky. Sid got The Scale from the Maltese Falcon. But how the Maltese Falcon got The Scale is shrouded in the mists of time.

The only requirement for using The Scale was to tip Pearl Toledo, Harry's wife. From this came the ancient adage for weighing yourself, Tippin the Toledos.

I'm sorry to tell you there is no more Magic Scale. It was stolen one night by the Apache Indians to weigh their chief, Fat Whispering Belly Button, and hasn't been seen since.

Scales and Cooking Equipment

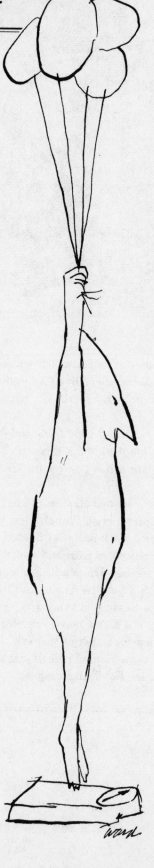

TERRAILLON CORPORATION
**95Q South Hoffman Lane
Central Islip, New York 11722**

Terraillon manufactures bathroom scales and other products that are so beautifully designed that some of them have been chosen for the permanent design collection of the Museum of Modern Art in New York.

Their model 111A bathroom scale is part of that collection, and it is a handsome devil. Suggested retail price is only $35, and you may buy it in blue, red, tangerine, white, or yellow. Just remember, regardless of how good-looking your bathroom scale is, it never looks prettier than when that needle dances to a lower number.

Terraillon sells eight other models, in all shapes, sizes, and colors, ranging in price from $16 to $39. They also give a lifelong guarantee on their bathroom scales for accuracy and reliability.

They also manufacture a diet scale which weighs up to one pound in quarter-ounce divisions, with a separate tray for liquids. This food scale retails for $14. And, for all you folks who like to mess around and make your own yogurt, they have a yogurt maker for $28.

You can find Terraillon products in better department stores. If not, write them at the above address.

CONTINENTAL SCALE CORPORATION
**Makers of Health-o-meter Bathroom and
  Doctor's Scales**
7400 West 100th Place
Bridgeview, Illinois 60455

A shiver went up my spine when I opened the big envelope from Continental Scale Corporation. I love scales, and the literature in the envelope was an orgy for my jaded number-ridden eyes. I—who've spent hours in houseware departments caressing scales—couldn't have been happier. This was nirvana. I hadn't been that excited since I was nine years old and got my Little Orphan Annie Secret Bombsight.

Health-o-meter calls itself "America's Weight-Watcher Since 1919." Now I know why. Their incredible supply of scales is sold at mass merchandisers, department stores, and surgical and hospital supply dealers.

I'll start off by telling you about the scale I'm going to save my pennies for: Doctor-Clinic/Beam Scale, model number 250. This is a doctor's-type scale without the high price. It is precisely graduated in quarter-pound units, up to a 300-pound capacity. Compact, lightweight, it fits easily in most bathrooms or bedrooms. And it has gliding adjustments and a waist-high slanted beam.

Then there is the Doctor Clinic Dial Scale—model 130: waist-high speedometer dial scale with 300-pound capacity for professional use with accuracy to the half-pound.

And finally, the Portable Scale—model 134: the rich, satin-finished carrying handle on this lightweight portable floor-model scale provides easy maneuverability. (That's what the catalog says, anyway.) Although it's not as compact as the dream scale I have invented for myself, it's the closest to an ideal portable scale that I know about.

Health-o-meter manufactures scales for every decor and need, in every color and material. Some are quilted, some are oval, some have both pound and kilo dials, some are rectangular, some are covered in fake fur, and some are so fancy you can keep them in your living room.

If you're really rich, you can indulge in the crème de la crème: the electronic scale with the digital readout made for the medical profession. Choose any one of the eight in the model 500 series.

Take your time. Pick out a scale you can live and be happy with. A scale for us diet people is nothing to trifle with. Check out the prices at your local store.

115

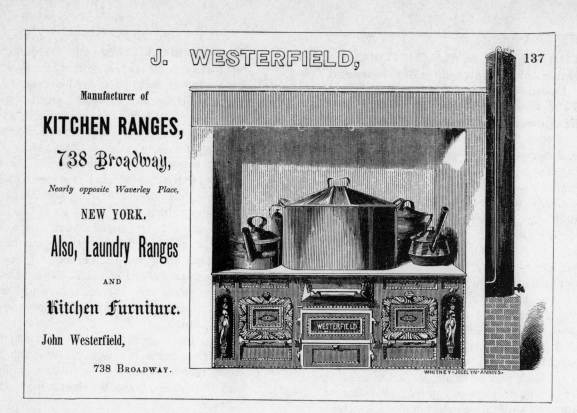

VITA MIX CORPORATION
8615 Usher Road
Cleveland, Ohio 44138

The Vita Mix machine grinds grain, mixes and kneads dough in one four-minute operation. Fresh fruit and vegetable juices can be made with whole fruits and vegetables. You can also throw in the skin, seeds, stem—everything—for added vitamins and low calories.

This item also mixes, grinds, grates, purees, liquefies, and makes baby food. It will chop meat, vegetables, and ice without the addition of any liquid. A pressurized serving spigot allows you to taste-test while you're mixing.

This thing will probably clean your house, if you ask it nicely.

With the Vita Mix 3600, a 130-page book of recipes is included. Suggested retail price is under $200. You can get one at your favorite department store or you may order direct from the company at the above address.

SALTON, INC. PRODUCTS
At your favorite store

SALTON AUTOMATIC EGG COOKER/
POACHER

The Salton Egg Cooker makes 'em poached or boiled for you. I don't have to tell you how many calories you save if you poach or boil your eggs rather than fix them scrambled or fried in butter, and this little machine takes the pain out of making boiled or poached eggs (I don't think I've ever gotten all the little pieces of shells out of my boiled eggs). With this Egg Cooker, you just add water and select the dial setting for soft, medium, hard, or anywhere in between. When the red light goes on the eggs are ready. So boil your calories away. Price is about $30.

SALTON YOGURT MAKER

The Salton Yogurt Maker makes one quart of yogurt using either skim or whole milk—add a tablespoon of yogurt and the Yogurt Maker does the rest. For a little something extra, they suggest adding your own natural fruit or other stuff. You'll save about seventy percent of the cost of commercial yogurt. Sells for about $13.

Exercise Equipment

BEACON ENTERPRISES INC.
230 Fifth Avenue
New York, New York 10001

Beacon Enterprises produces popular-priced fitness equipment for the home. Their products are sold in major department stores and discount houses.

You can trim down with exercise boards, bicycle exercisers, special devices for legs, tummy, and bust, and rowing machines.

I notice that all the models in the catalog are women except one. Why didn't they ask me to be the lucky man?

DIVERSIFIED PRODUCTS
CORPORATION
309 Williamson Avenue
Opelika, Alabama 36801

Diversified is sure the right name for Diversified Products. They put out a whole slew of physical fitness equipment described in detail in their catalog.

There are barbells for men, women, and children in every conceivable size and variety. There are solid dumbells for men and women, exercise benches, the famous Exer-Gym used by the Apollo astronauts, exercise bicycles, jump ropes, chest pulls, chinning bars and a complete home gym.

Every time I read one of these fitness catalogs and see those pictures of the muscular models, I figure, hell, I'm going to look like that soon. But it hasn't happened yet. I guess you have to buy the equipment and use it. Darn.

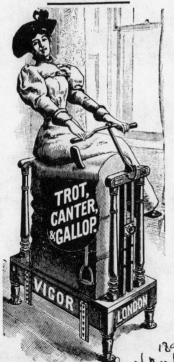

MARGRACE CORPORATION
201 Lincoln Boulevard
Middlesex, New Jersey 08846

Send for free brochure describing these items:

BULLWORKER 3

An isometric exerciser with a built-in Powermeter. Each exercise takes just a few seconds a day. Margrace says you can increase your strength up to four percent a week, and also reduce your stomach measurements, with the Bullworker.

BULLWORKER FLEXERCISER

A flexible spring-tension exerciser which is available in three different tensions, for men, women, and children.

BULLWORKER CRUSHER

A dual-purpose body-builder for pushing and pulling exercises. There are eight degrees of tensions—you can choose.

EVANS PRECISION, INC.
P.O. Box 366
Lancaster, Ohio 43130

DYNA-BAR

Evans Precision says, "Dyna-Bar is the new and different approach to in-the-home body development and weight-trimming for all ages—men, women and children." It uses isometric contraction to strengthen muscles.

FORMIDABLE EXERCISER

This is a pulley device that's supposed to tone muscles and trim inches. The whole exerciser attaches to any doorknob.

BODY TONER JUMP ROPE

You get two things for one here—it's a jump rope and, if you adjust the rope and handles, an isometric exerciser.

Check your sporting goods store, department store, or discount house for these items. If you can't find them, write to Evans at the above address.

New York City's building laws require a 19-inch-width minimum for theater seats. For a person who weighs upward of 270 pounds and stands 5 feet 11 inches tall, with a standing backside spread of about 21 inches, which expands under compression, the overflow must go over the arm of the seat or, somehow, forward. Which makes for a pretty tight fit.

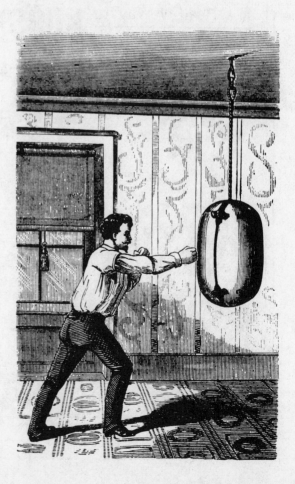

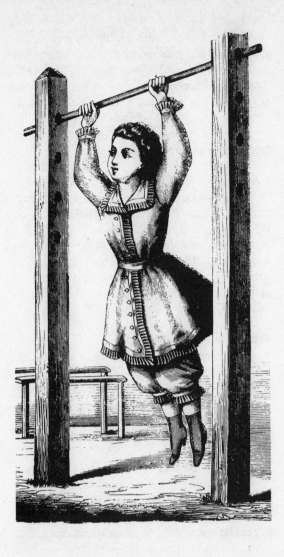

Whitely puts out just the equipment to help take off inches, provided you exercise regularly.

There are four different varieties of Home Gyms, depending on your needs. You can work up a real sweat with hand grippers, chest pulls, jump ropes, tone wheels for your tummy, and attachments for wall pulls.

Whitely also offers a travel gym, an isometric exercise kit, Jiffy Gyms, seven different kinds of jump ropes, barbells, exercise benches, mats, and exercise bicycles.

Get off those lazy buns of yours. It's time to get in shape. You're losing weight, now tighten up that flab. This company has many products that may help.

Wonder makes exercise bikes, tennis trainers, rower exercisers, chest developers, hand grips, gym bars, jump ropes, family fitness exercise sets, slantboards, mats, exercise wheels, and exercise benches.

Check your local stores. If they don't have what you want, write Wonder for the store nearest you.

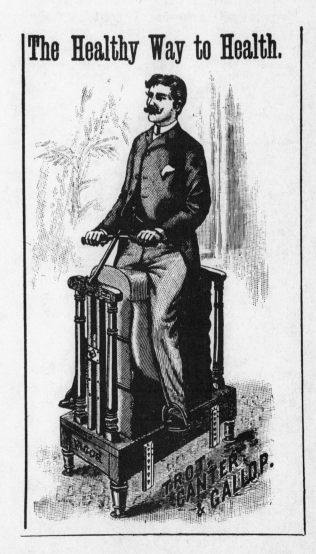

The Healthy Way to Health.

WALTON MANUFACTURING COMPANY
106 Regal Row
Dallas, Texas 75247

"Our equipment is not sold for weight reduction but is for exercise to be used in conjunction with a diet program for those who wish to lose weight," says this company. Right up front they tell you to cut down on the groceries, along with using their exercise equipment, if you want to take off those pounds.

ROWABOUT $139.50
From their brochure: "Rowing has long been considered an excellent means of strengthening major muscle groups, including shoulders, thighs, back, chest, arms, ankles, wrists and stomach. Endurance and stamina may be improved as well."

STATIONARY BIKES
Walton offers three models of stationary bikes, ranging in price from $99.50 to $124.50.

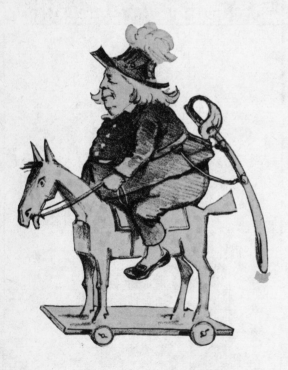

All of them have various controls to adjust pedaling resistance, speedometer-odometer, and cushioned seat with quick height adjustment. There are differences in construction and other points, but the best model has an exclusive feature—a swiveling handlebar action which lets you do swimming-type exercises for the upper body while you're pedaling.

CAROUSEL JOGGER
This is designed to duplicate running, walking, or jogging with foot platforms in an up, down, and around motion. Free-swing handlebars complement natural body and arm movement. There's a balanced flywheel to maintain momentum and desired speed and a speedometer-odometer gauge. The price is $189.50.

TREADMILL JOGGERS
Walk, run, or jog with either of two models costing $199.50 and $299.50. Both have hardwood rollers with a pedometer to measure each day's workout. The more expensive jogger has sidebars, is better constructed, and is adjustable for flat or inclined use.

ELECTRIC CYCLES
These electric-driven cycles offer a wide range of exercises. The exercise programs can vary from "very little" to "strenuous" depending on how you adjust the speed-control knob. You can have simulated swimming, rowing, cycling, and riding exercises. There are two different models, offering single-speed or variable speed. The prices are $299.50 and $369.50.

The advantage of these machines is, of course, that you're not dependent on the whims of Mother Nature. Muggers won't chase you, dogs won't nip at your heels, and you won't step in any little presents that the doggies leave behind.

Writing about all this exercise equipment has made me feel very fit—and also very exhausted. I'm going to lie down now.

Diet clothes

This is an important consideration for people on diets. What do you do for clothes? Women seem to have it a little easier than men in this. They can wear tent dresses and loose-fitting blouses and skirts until they get down. But men's clothes tend to be more tailored and closer fitting; if they don't fit fairly well, they look a mess. There's not much a man can do about the situation unless he's got a tub full of money and can afford different-size wardrobes as needed.

I don't have so much of a problem because I've never been much of a clothes person. Just give me a shirt, a pair of Levi's, sweat socks, and saddle shoes and I'll go anywhere. When I was coming down in weight, I just let my clothes get baggy. I once had a date who told me that I must spend all of twenty dollars a year on clothes. Actually, I was flattered—I probably average about ten dollars a year.

Anyway, whether you're a man or a woman, if you're taking off large amounts of weight (unless you have large amounts of money), you're going to have a clothing problem. So, unless you're handy with a sewing machine or your brother-in-law's a tailor, just say the hell with it—weight is a more serious problem than clothes, and the best-fitting clothes in the world won't look good if you're overweight. Just try to hold off until you get to your ideal weight, then go out and buy lots of new clothes. Your new duds could be a great incentive to stay down where you belong.

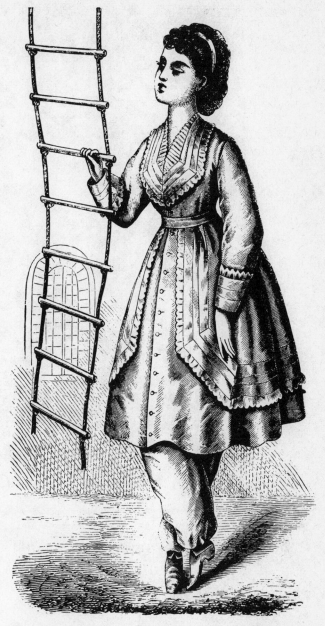

GYMNASTIC SUIT FOR GIRL FROM 10 TO 12 YEARS OLD.

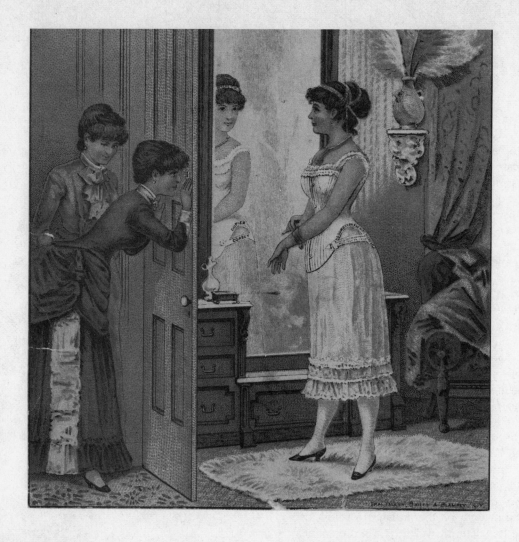

HOW TO MAKE CLOTHES THAT FIT AND FLATTER
by Adele P. Margolis
$7.95 Hardbound 296 pages
Doubleday

For all you women who need to alter your clothes as you shed those pounds, or who'd like to make new clothes for the new you, this could be the book.

How to Make Clothes contains easy-to-follow directions, copious how-to drawings, and many styling tips. Ms. Margolis is a well-known sewing teacher and says that, with this book, the art of fitting can be attained by every sewer.

Since I have to hire someone to sew on a button, sewing is not my thing. But if you like to thread that bobbin and tote that pattern, this book could save you lots of money—and maybe make you look like a fairy princess.

BUTTERICK PATTERN SERVICE
161 Sixth Avenue
New York, New York 10013
London Toronto Sydney

The Butterick Pattern people offer several flattering patterns for those women who are overweight and those who are overweight and hopefully on the way down.

They've given them a great name: Butterick Seams Slimmer. I've never used a sewing machine or a pattern, but they look terrific to me. Take a look and judge for yourself.

The patterns run from $1.25 to $1.50, slightly higher in Canada.

If you need to travel before you take those pounds off, it might help you to know how much room you'll get in which kinds of airplanes. For most airlines, the DC-10 allows 21 inches in first class, 18.3 inches in coach. The DC-8 has 22.7 inches in first, 16.8 inches in coach. The 747 has 21 or 22 inches in first, 18.3 inches in coach. The 727 is one of the narrowest: 19.9 inches in first, 16.5 in coach. In most coach seating, a well-rounded person must squeeze to make room for the dining tray to lie flat in front of him. Makes you think.

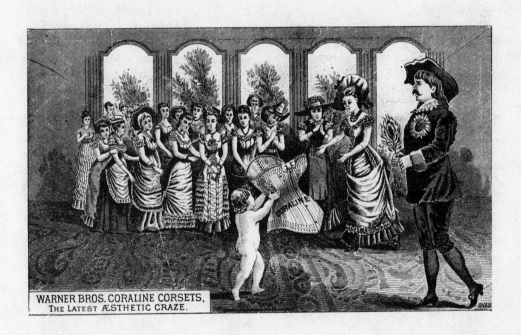

WARNER BROS. CORALINE CORSETS,
The Latest Æsthetic Craze.

Records, Tapes, & Cassettes

SMI, INC.
5000 Lakewood Drive
Waco, Texas 76710
Phone: (817) 776-1230
Makers of the Listen and Succeed
  Cassette Tape Series

According to the brochure for the cassette tape "Listen and Lose," by Dr. Robert Parrish, "To lose weight our subconscious must visualize us as being slim. Otherwise, it will wreck any conscious diet! Listen and Lose will help you reach your subconscious with a slim image. Before you know it, you will act slim, be slim, and stay that way, without dieting."

If you want the cassette, send $9.95 plus 20¢ postage to the above address.

This could be a revolutionary way to lose weight through the ears. There certainly is a lot of fat between my ears.

EDWIN L. BARON, Ph.D.
116 South Michigan Avenue
Chicago, Illinois 60603

Edwin L. Baron bills himself as "Master Hypnotist." He specializes in hypnosis to help you lose weight, and he has made a record called "Reduce Through Listening." This is a special double-life record based on therapeutic principles of subconscious re-education; it helps you to listen away your undesirable eating habits through reinforced suggestions. It conditions you to avoid high-calorie foods and liquids and to prefer and desire low-calorie foods and liquids until you reach the weight you wish.

You may write for the record to the Baronette Recording Company at the above address.

The cost of the record is $6.95; as a cassette, $7.95. Tax (outside of Illinois) and prepaid mailing costs are included.

1, 2, 3, 4. 1, 2, 3, 4. 1, 2, 3, 4.

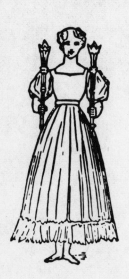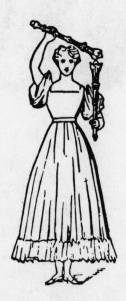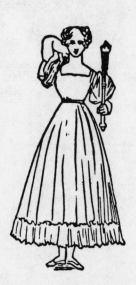

FEEL GOOD! LOOK GREAT!
Exercise Along with Debbie Drake
With Noel Regency and His Orchestra
Epic Records

All right, twinkle-toes—now all you would-be Gene Kellys, Fred Astaires, Leslie Carons, and Cyd Charisses can exercise to twist tunes and waltz melodies and, of course, your leader, Debbie Drake.

There are nineteen exercises on this album, each of them set to two different pieces of music for variety's sake. Ms. Drake says to exercise fifteen minutes a day, preferably in the morning. I don't think in those nineteen exercises there is one tiny little muscle that Debbie doesn't work on.

Included with the record is a helpful booklet with a calorie-counter, "Debbie Drake's Diet Tips," and photographs showing how to do all the exercises.

She also suggests you exercise with a friend for more fun. I couldn't agree more. Could be a way to meet new people. I think I'll go next door and ask one of the stewardesses to come over for a workout.

HOW TO KEEP YOUR HUSBAND HAPPY
Look Slim! Keep Trim! Exercise Along With Debbie Drake
Original Music Composed and Conducted by Frank Hunter

"Do you know that overweight is a threat to the happiest of marriages?" asks Debbie Drake. She tells us that if you diet and follow the exercises in this album, you'll have a figure desired by men and envied by women. Every part of the body, even the hands and feet, will be exercised.

The record comes with a booklet illustrating all the exercises in photographs, so it's easy for you to follow. The photographs of Ms. Drake doing the exercises show that she practices what she preaches. If a woman will look like Debbie Drake after dieting and doing the exercises, then this record should become the best-selling album of all time.

1, 2, 3, 4. 1, 2, 3, 4. 1, 2, 3, 4.

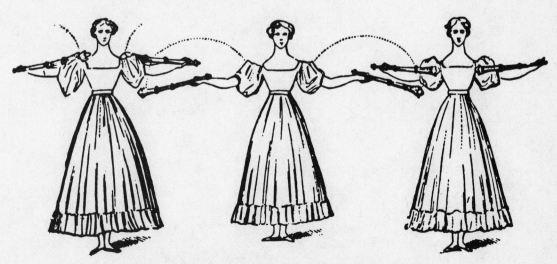

EXERCISES WITH INDIAN SCEPTERS

Godey's Lady's Book, 1849.

FOUR

IN COMPANY

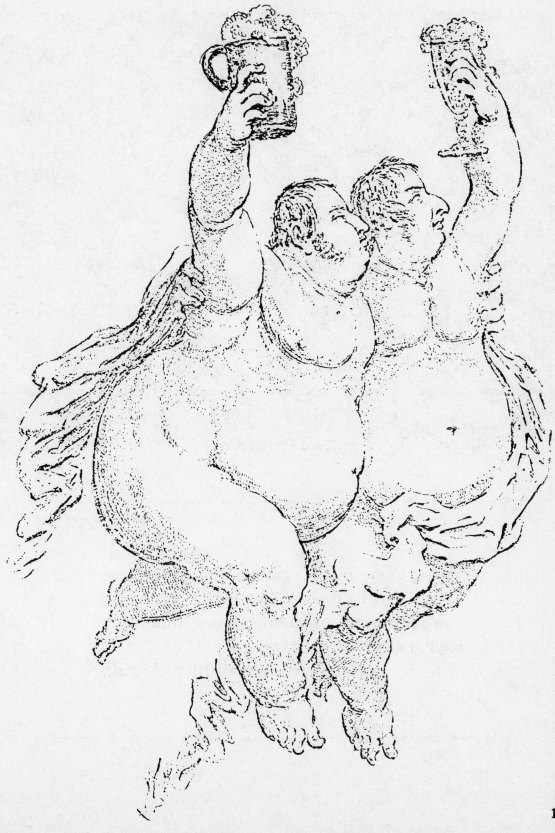

Diet Groups

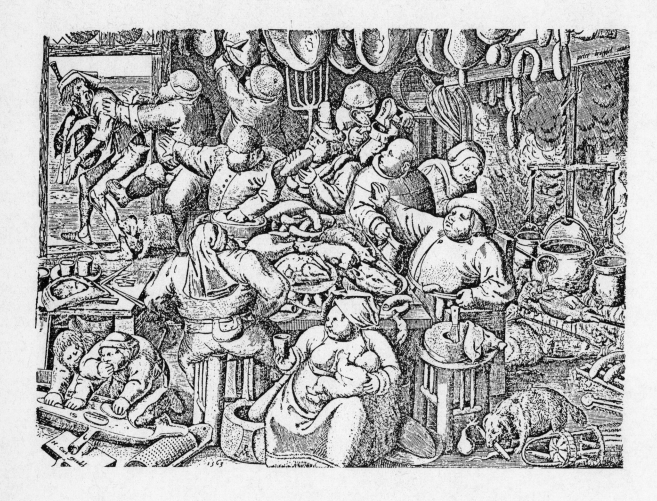

"Eating alone fosters egotism, encourages one
to care only for oneself, isolates one from
one's surroundings, dissuades one from
paying little polite attentions. . . ."
—Anthelme Brillat-Savarin

I think diet groups are terrific. They're the best thing to happen to dieting since the bikini. My only regret is that when I started dieting seventeen years ago, there were none around for me to join. At least I couldn't find any. So I had to go it alone. And believe me, it *was* lonely.

The group support, the sharing of experiences, the wealth of sound diet information these organizations have available to them—all these factors make losing weight easier in a group. But remember, you still have to go it alone most of the time. No one is going to be standing next to you every time you're eyeballing an apricot Danish in the bakery window. But there are groups that work on the buddy system. You can call a diet buddy for help if that Danish is about to leap out of the window and into your mouth.

There are many groups and almost all of them cost money. With the variety of groups and individual plans, I'm sure everyone can find one to help him or her.

Talk to friends about their experiences, write or call a number of groups, look at the available brochures, attend free introductory meetings if any are offered in your area. Just be careful to find a group *you* feel comfortable with.

National

WEIGHT WATCHERS INTERNATIONAL, INC.
800 Community Drive
Manhasset, New York 11030
Phone: (516) 627-9200

Unless you've been living in the bottom of a strawberry cheesecake for the last couple of decades, you must have heard of Weight Watchers.

It's the General Motors of the dieting world, with classes being held over much of the world. More than eight million people have enrolled in W.W. and every week there are approximately 12,000 individual classes held around the globe. No more boring statistics. Let's just say that Weight Watchers is big and that they've been hugely successful in helping a great many people lose weight. Very, very briefly let me tell you what W.W. is all about.

Jean Nidetch, founder of Weight Watchers, and her staff have developed the following program to help the overweight. You must be at least ten pounds overweight to join. Weight Watchers' purpose is to re-educate your eating habits so that you can learn to keep the weight off forever. There are three steps to their program:

1. The Basic Plan: teaches you how to satisfy your appetite with the right foods and moves you steadily toward your goal weight.
2. The Leveling Plan: helps you through the last ten pounds from your goal weight and prepares you for the Maintenance Plan.
3. The Maintenance Plan: you can gradually add to your diet all of your favorites, in proper quantities, that you had to give up while achieving goal weight, without putting the weight back on again.

But there's much more to Weight Watchers than those weekly meetings. There's *Weight Watchers Magazine; Weight Watchers Program Cookbook; The Story of Weight Watchers,* which is an autobiography of Jean

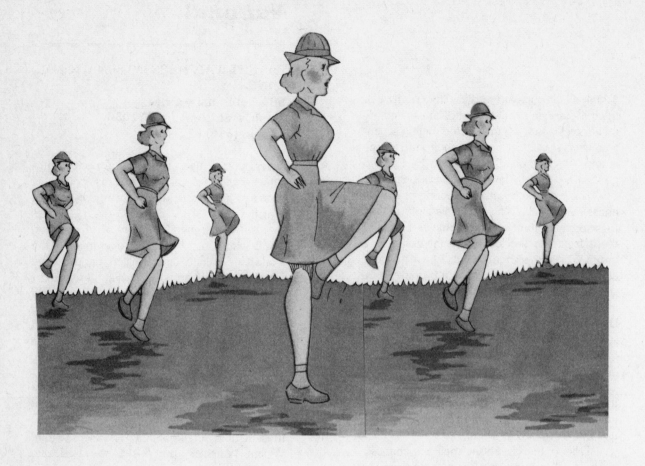

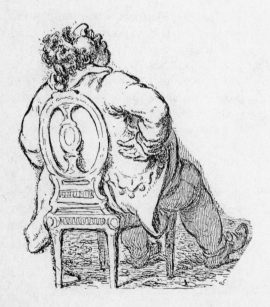

Nidetch; *Ask Jean,* a collection of letters that have been written to Jean Nidetch. There are two companies putting out special W.W. foods, and licensed Weight Watchers camps for overweight boys and girls. With their fantastic growth, maybe Weight Watchers can bail out New York.

If you're interested in W.W., look them up in your local phone book and go to a meeting. They're probably anywhere where there's indoor plumbing.

Weight Watchers is a franchise business and costs vary from area to area. They charge a modest registration fee, usually between three and five dollars. The regular weekly meeting fee runs from two to four dollars.

THE DIET WORKSHOP, INC.
1975 Hempstead Turnpike
East Meadow, New York 11554
Phone: (516) 794-4881

Diet Workshops are one of the biggies in the weight-reduction biz. They are the second largest national chain of franchised group weight-control programs. You know which one is first. There are now sixty-four Diet Workshops in thirty-one states, Canada, and Bermuda, with over 1400 groups containing approximately 45,000 people meeting weekly.

Diet Workshops were started in 1965 by two overweight housewives, Lois Lindauer and Edith Berman, in Boston, Massachusetts. Ms. Lindauer is now the National Director and Ms. Berman is Director of Research and Development.

The diet itself is a 1200-calorie, measured-portion, three-meal-a-day balanced diet. You must eat from the basic four food groups every day to assure nutritional balance. There are also hints and tips on between-meal nibbles, snacks, and drinks. Creative diet cooking is encouraged and a new recipe is dictated to each class every week. Dr. Morton Glenn became Nutritional Consultant to The Diet Workshop in 1968 and developed the present diet.

In 1975, a behavioral modification program was added to nutrition and diet as one of the methods of successful weight control. Each week on a six-week cycle, a new method of eating behavior is called for. Through the six-week cycle of simple steps, dieters learn the relationship between the manner of eating, the reason for eating, and resultant overweight.

All members are given a great deal of individual attention. If a member drops out before reaching his goal weight, he is called and asked to come back.

After the member reaches goal weight, four weeks' free maintenance instruction is given. Then the member becomes a free lifetime member. He may attend classes free as long as he remains within two pounds of his goal weight. All lifetime members are encouraged to come in once a month for a weigh-in. I guess you can say, Diet Workshop cares.

The charge for the first meeting is six dollars; for each meeting after that, two dollars and fifty cents.

The Diet Workshop motto is: "It's In to Be Thin." If you're into being thin, get those fat little fingers of yours moving and look up the nearest Diet Workshop in the White or Yellow Pages, or write to the above address for the Diet Workshop nearest you.

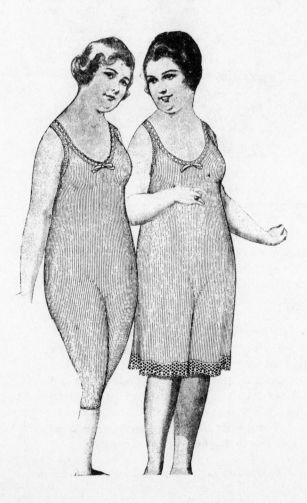

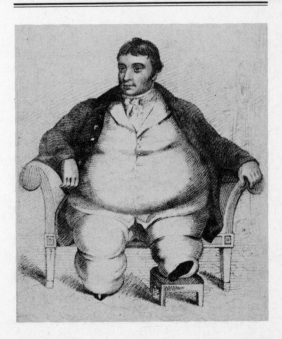

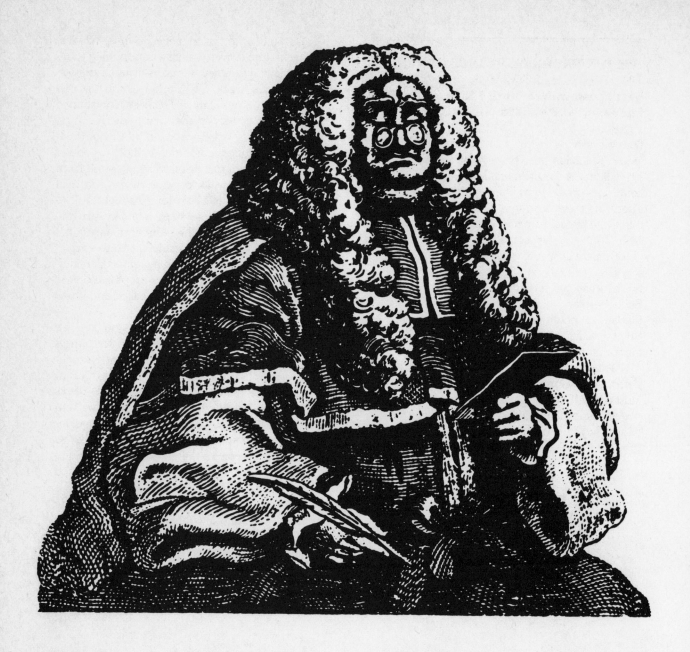

MOVIE

A MATTER OF FAT
National Film Board of Canada
1251 Avenue of the Americas, New York,
** New York 10020**
16 mm.   99 minutes   Color. $850;
** $85 (rental)**

I haven't seen this movie but I sure would like to. This was the only movie I could find that dealt with obesity and weight control.

According to the catalog, *A Matter of Fat* portrays a 357-pound man losing 140 pounds in a hospital fasting program. Also there's a panorama of what is considered fat—from the glamorous society woman's excess ounces to a 700-pound carnival fat lady. A teen diet camp, a TOPS convention, a Weight Watchers meeting and diet frauds and dangers are also shown and explored.

As the catalog says; "Anyone concerned with obesity will be moved and informed by this film."

Sorry, kids, no hot buttered popcorn permitted in the theater.

OVEREATERS ANONYMOUS/WORLD SERVICE OFFICE
3730 Motor Avenue
Los Angeles, California 90034
Phone: (213) 559-6140

Overeaters Anonymous is not a diet group but a fellowship of men and women who meet and share their experiences to "recover from the disease of compulsive overeating."

O.A. is a nonprofit organization with over 1400 groups meeting in the U.S. The program was started by three Los Angeles housewives in 1960 who patterned O.A. after Alcoholics Anonymous and Gamblers Anonymous.

Overeaters Anonymous can best be described from their own letter:

"We believe that we have a progressive, three-fold illness affecting us physically, emotionally and spiritually. Over a considerable length of time it gets worse, never better. There are no dues or fees for O.A. membership. We are self-supporting through our own contributions—the basket is passed during each meeting.

"How does it work? We treat the emotional and spiritual portions of our problem by following the Twelve Steps, Twelve Traditions and principles of the Alcoholics Anonymous program. We learn the tools to use, so that no matter what comes to us in life we do not have to eat to avoid our problems.

"In responding to physical manifestations of our illness, many of us believe that we have a sensitivity to refined sugars and flour. One bite leads to another . . . another. Therefore, Overeaters Anonymous has two *suggested* eating plans for losing weight. Each is a disciplined manner of eating three weighed and measured meals a day with nothing in between except black coffee, tea or sugar-free beverages— each calls for total abstinence from refined sugars and flour. They both work! We also have a plan for maintaining weight loss."

O.A. does not recommend any one particular diet. O.A. also advises you to see your doctor for your particular calorie and nutrient needs.

I attended an Overeaters Anonymous meeting about six years ago with a friend who was doing a newspaper story about the O.A. program. What impressed me was the depth of the involvement by the people in the group. Only first names were used, preserving anonymity. I was a little scared at first by the outpouring of problems, hurts, and fears that all of us obese and formerly obese have experienced, but that I had never before heard exposed. After a while these fears left, because of all the help people were receiving in the group. The people I know in O.A. are totally dedicated to the program and it works for them on all levels.

For more information, look in your phone book or else write Overeaters Anonymous at the above address.

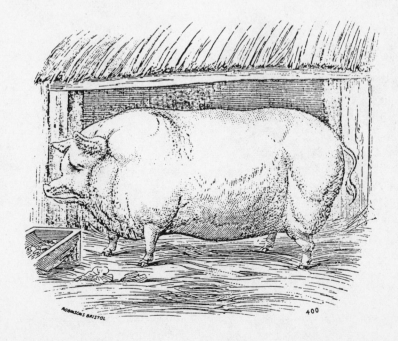

The East

APPETITE CONTROL CENTERS
P.O. Box 268
Hopewell Junction, New York 12533
Phone: (914) 226-4745

How would you like to go on a diet where you can have mayonnaise, potatoes, rice, macaroni, spaghetti, desserts, and shakes? You're all excited and you're salivating like the Colorado River. Well, you can have these in limited amounts on Appetite Control Centers' diet.

They have 100 groups in New York State, Pennsylvania, and Connecticut. Linda Mayer, the founder, lost her weight on the New York City Board of Health Weight Reducing Diet.

She writes a weekly column that runs in thirty newspapers.

There are weekly meetings where you are re-educated to eat properly and lose weight at the same time. Once you've reached your goal, you then go on a maintenance program.

Appetite Control Centers charge six dollars for the first week and three dollars per week thereafter; half price for families and senior citizens. There are also reduced-rate plans for all members.

By the way, they're approved by the New York State Board of Education to give nutritional guidance.

VANTILE MACK, THE INFANT LAMBERT, OR
GIANT BABY!!
7 Years old. Weighs 257 pounds!
Measures 61 inches around the chest!! 36 inches around the leg!!
With his Mother, only 21 years of age.
NOW EXHIBITING AT BARNUM'S AMERICAN MUSEUM.

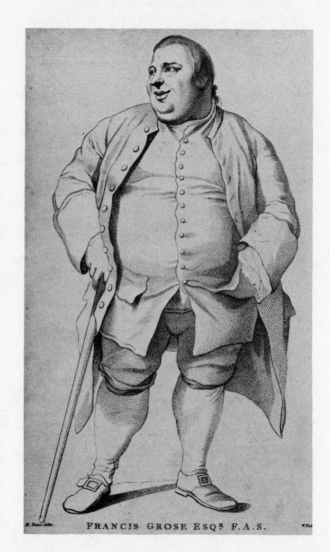

FRANCIS GROSE ESQ? F.A.S.

DIET CONTROL CENTERS, INC.
1021 Stuyvesant Avenue
Union, New Jersey 07083
Phone: (201) 687-0007
In Manhattan call (212) 734-9060

Diet Control Centers are diet groups that use a diet based on that of the New York City Health Department, jazzing it up with ethnic foods and more variety. (Maybe they could invent a lo-cal egg roll.) For all the details of the Diet Control Centers look under *Slim Forever—The Diet Control Centers Diet* (see above, page 11).

The Diet Control groups charge dues and registration fees. They advise you to follow your doctor's advice and, if required by state law, to submit a doctor's certificate before joining. You can attend as many meetings weekly as desired at no extra charge after paying the initial weekly fee. If you're hot for meetings, this could be the ticket.

After reaching "Control Weight," there are four weekly steps in which you may add certain foods to your diet. At the end of the four weeks you become a Lifetime Control Member. You can then attend weekly meetings free, as long as you don't exceed your goal weight. In plain English, if you balloon up again, you have to pay weekly dues again, but you don't have to pay a re-registration fee.

Behavioral modification, a fairly new tool in the overthrow of obesity, has been introduced recently in Diet Control Centers. With behavior mod, reducers record their every bite in diaries so they can see their eating patterns and correct them if necessary.

Diet Control Centers also publish several recipe books and a bimonthly newspaper for you to read while your fat drops off.

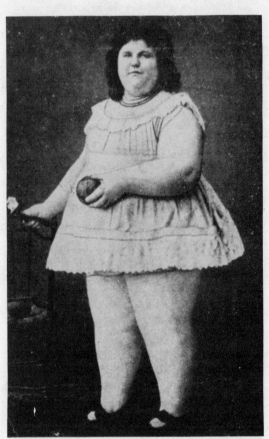

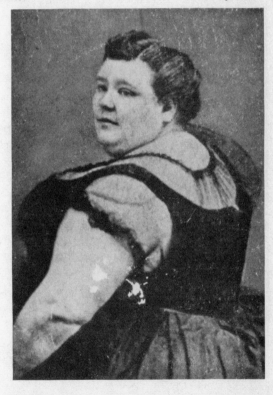

La colosse russe.   Jenny LETTO.

"Her waist is ampler than her life, for life is but a span."
—Oliver Wendell Holmes

THE NEW YORK CITY DEPARTMENT OF HEALTH DIET

You may drink

Coffee	Water	Bouillon
Tea	Club soda	Consommé

You may use

Salt	Herbs	Lemon, Lime
Pepper	Spices	Vinegar
	Horseradish	

You may eat freely

Asparagus	Cucumber	Romaine
Green Beans	Dandelion	Lettuce
Broccoli	Greens	Spinach
Brussels	Escarole	Summer Squash
Sprouts	Kale	Swiss Chard
Carrots	Lettuce	Tomato
Cauliflower	Mushrooms	Turnip Greens
Celery	Mustard	Watercress
Chicory	Greens	
Collards	Parsley	

You may not eat or drink

Bacon, Fatty Meats, Sausage
Beer, Liquor, Wines
Butter, Margarines other than de- scribed at right
Cakes, Cookies, Crackers, Doughnuts, Pastries, Pies
Candy, Chocolates, Nuts
Cream—Sweet and Sour, Cream Cheese, Non-Dairy Cream Substitutes
French Fried Potatoes, Potato Chips
Pizza, Popcorn, Pretzels and Similar Snack Foods

Gelatin Desserts, Puddings (sugar- sweetened)
Gravies and Sauces
Honey, Jams, Jellies Sugar and Syrup
Ice Cream, Ices, Ice Milk, Sherbets
Milk, Whole
Muffins, Pancakes, Waffles
Olives
Soda (sugar-sweetened)
Yogurt (fruit-flavored)

FOOD GROUPS

1. Limit these protein foods
   Lean beef, pork, lamb to 1 pound per week total
   Eggs to 4 per week
   Hard cheese to 4 oz. per week·

2. High Vitamin C fruits *(No added sugar)*

1 medium Orange	4 oz. Orange or
½ medium Canta- loupe	Grapefruit Juice
	½ medium Grapefruit
1 cup Strawberries	1 large Tangerine
½ medium Mango	8 oz. Tomato Juice

3. Other fruits *(No added sugar)*

1 medium Apple or Peach	2–3 Apricots, Prunes or Plums
1 small Banana or Pear	½ round slice Watermelon (1" by 10")
¼ lb. Cherries or Grapes	
½ cup Pineapple	½ small Honeydew Melon
½ cup Berries	2 Tablespoons Raisins

4. High Vitamin A vegetables

Broccoli	Mustard	Spinach
Carrots	greens,	Watercress
Chicory	Collards,	Escarole
Pumpkin,	and other	
Winter	leafy greens	
Squash		

5. Potato or substitute

1 medium Potato	½ cup Corn or green
1 small Sweet Potato or Yam	Lima Beans, Peas
1 small ear Corn	½ cup cooked dry Beans, Peas, Lentils
½ cup cooked Rice, Spaghetti, Macaroni, Grits or Noodles	
½ cup Plantain, Ñame or Yautía	

6. Fat

1 teaspoon Vege- table Oil	1 teaspoon Margarine with liquid vegetable oil listed first on label of ingredients
1 teaspoon Mayon- naise	
2 teaspoons French Dressing	

7. Skim milk or substitute
   2 cups (8 oz. each) Buttermilk
   1 cup (8 oz.) Evaporated Skimmed Milk
   ⅔ cup nonfat Dry Milk Solids

FOR MOST WOMEN AND SMALL FRAME MEN
Your 1200-Calorie Menu Plan

Breakfast
High Vitamin C Fruit
  Choose ONE from Group 2
Protein Food—Choose ONE:
  2 oz. cottage or pot cheese
  1 oz. hard cheese
  2 oz. cooked or canned fish
  1 egg
  8 oz. cup skimmed milk
Bread or Cereal, whole grain or enriched—Choose ONE:
  1 slice bread
  ¾ cup ready-to-eat cereal
  ½ cup cooked cereal
Coffee or tea

Lunch
Protein Food—Choose ONE:
  2 oz. fish, poultry or lean meat
  4 oz. cottage or pot cheese
  2 oz. hard cheese
  1 egg
  2 level tablespoons peanut butter
Bread—whole grain or enriched—2 slices
Vegetables—raw or cooked—except potato or substitute
Fruit—1 serving
Coffee or Tea

Dinner
Protein Food—Choose ONE:
  4 oz. cooked fish, poultry or lean meat
Vegetables cooked and raw
  High Vitamin A—Choose from Group 4
  Potato or substitute—Choose ONE from Group 5
  Other vegetables—you may eat freely
Fruit—1 serving
Coffee or Tea

Other daily foods
Fat—Choose 3 from Group 6
Milk—2 cups (8 oz. each) skimmed or substitute from Group 7

FOR MOST MEN AND LARGE FRAME WOMEN
Your 1600-Calorie Menu Plan

Breakfast
High Vitamin C Fruit
  Choose ONE from Group 2
Protein Food—Choose ONE:
  2 oz. cottage or pot cheese
  1 oz. hard cheese
  2 oz. cooked or canned fish
  1 egg
  8 oz. cup skimmed milk
Bread or Cereal, whole grain or enriched—Choose ONE:
  2 slices bread
  1½ cups ready-to-eat cereal
  1 cup cooked cereal
Coffee or Tea

Lunch
Protein Food—Choose ONE:
  2 oz. fish, poultry or lean meat
  4 oz. cottage or pot cheese
  2 oz. hard cheese
  1 egg
  2 level tablespoons peanut butter
Bread—whole grain or enriched—2 slices
Vegetables—raw or cooked—except potato or substitute
Fruit—1 serving
Coffee or Tea

Dinner
Protein Food—Choose ONE:
  6 oz. cooked fish, poultry or lean meat
Vegetables—raw and cooked
  High Vitamin A—Choose from Group 4
  Potato or Substitute—Choose ONE from Group 5
  Other vegetables—you may eat freely
Fruit—1 serving
Coffee or Tea

Other daily foods
Fat—Choose 6 from Group 6
Milk—2 cups (8 oz. each) skimmed or substitute from Group 7

Since New York City cannot afford to mail this diet out to each and every one of you, and since this diet has been used as the basis for so many others, I decided to reproduce it for you, courtesy of the Bureau of Nutrition of the New York City Department of Health.

WHY WEIGHT? INC.
1424 Sheepshead Bay Road
Brooklyn, New York 11235
Phone: (212) 769-3737

Why Weight? was started twelve years ago by Sidney Goldstein, who lost 104 pounds. Now there are fifty-five groups throughout Brooklyn; they have helped over 150,000 Brooklynites get rid of excess pounds.

They use the original Dr. Norman Jolliffe diet from the New York City Health Department. Behavior modification is also used, so once you're slim you won't gain the weight back.

Why Weight? offers small classes for more personalized rapport, a telephone "hot line," free cooking classes, luncheons where awards for losing one hundred pounds and for other achievements are presented, and a free maintenance program. Why Weight? is registered with New York City Board of Health.

All of the classes are held in Brooklyn, New York. There's a Why Weight? program at The Jewish Hospital and Medical Center of Brooklyn for their staff and a program set up at Blue Cross and Blue Shield for their employees. Brooklyn must have a lot of good cooks and great restaurants to have all those overweight folks.

The cost of Why Weight? is four dollars for registration and three dollars for weekly dues.

If you live some place like Sioux City, Iowa, and want to go to Why Weight?, come on up and I'll rent you some living space on the Brooklyn Bridge cheap.

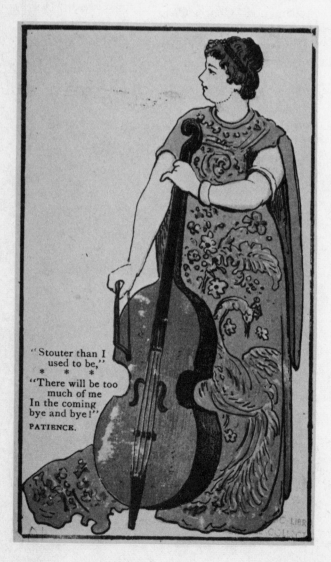

"Stouter than I
used to be,"
* * *
"There will be too
much of me
In the coming
bye and bye!"
PATIENCE.

WEIGH OF LIFE
430 West Merrick Road
Valley Stream, New York 11580
Phone: (516) 872-8181

Weigh of Life is a diet organization located primarily in the New York area. However, they hope to be in the Florida and Boston areas soon.

The diet itself is the New York City Health Department diet, with modifications. This means it's healthful and nutritious, and you may substitute different foods at each meal so you won't get bored. For instance, for the main course at breakfast you may choose among: one egg; one ounce hard cheese; two ounces fish; two ounces cottage, farmer, or pot cheese; or three-quarters cup dry cereal.

Weigh of Life uses a psychological approach to losing weight, too. Behavior modification principles are also used.

There are group meetings each week. The charge is seven dollars for the first meeting, which includes registration, and three dollars per week for weekly meetings thereafter. A member may drop out of a group at any time, but members will be charged three dollars for each meeting missed. You may have a two-week vacation period if you notify the clerk before starting the vacation. After your goal weight is reached, you may attend as many meetings as you want for free, if you stay within three pounds of your goal weight.

As Weigh of Life says:
Don't Put it Off.
Or You'll Put It On!

THE WEIGHT COUNCIL LTD.
New York, New York
Joel Grinker, Ph.D.
Phone: (212) 360-1694

Dr. Grinker has been associated with The Rockefeller University and their obesity research program for several years. His Weight Council uses behavioral modification and nutrition counseling to help people lose weight and keep it off.

You are given an extensive questionaire on past diets, how successful they were, family history, when, where, and how you eat, food preferences, and so forth.

Then you are asked to keep a diary of everything you eat for ten weeks. As the Weight Council points out: "In order to modify behavior, it is essential and imperative that all behaviors which are involved in the intake of food be carefully recorded and analyzed." This way you can look at your total eating behavior and habits, alter your behavior, and, it is hoped, be successful at weight reducing.

The following weeks are devoted to changing your eating behavior plus an intensive nutritional education.

The Weight Council course lasts ten weeks, and costs $175 plus a $5 registration fee.

LEAN LINE, INC.
1600 Park Avenue
South Plainfield, New Jersey 07080
Phone: (201) 757-7677

Lean Line's motto is "Mind over matter." In their brochure, a cartoon shows a woman's head with an arrow pointing to the middle of her forehead with the caption, "The smartest place to start a diet."

Ms. Lolly Wurtzel and Ms. Toni Marotta, two former Weight Watchers and the co-founders of Lean Line, use behavioral modifi-cation and a calorie diet as their basic plan to lose weight.

According to them, what makes Lean Line's program unique is its behavioral modification techniques. Here are some of them.

1. Forks should be put down on the plate after every bite of food and not picked up again until the food has been chewed and swallowed. This slows the overweight person down. Food is enjoyed more. You get fuller faster. Therefore you eat less. Sounds easy, doesn't it? Yours truly has tried this method for over five years and it works. But it's the toughest thing in the world for me to do. I want to keep shoveling faster and faster. Try it. It is the best piece of diet advice I've ever received.
2. As soon as you, the Lean Liner, finish eating, you should leave the table.
3. You cannot stand and eat—always sit down. At a table.
4. Your meals must be eaten at the same times and in the same place.
5. Small plates are to be used. This makes it look as if there's more food on your plate. Clever.
6. You may drink liquids after the meal only.
7. You must never go grocery-shopping on an empty stomach.

Besides the behavioral modification, there is a calorie diet. You can eat such things as spaghetti, sour cream, and pizza, but in very precise, measured amounts. What they have tried to do is balance the diet with a psychological balance.

Since Lean Line was started eight years ago, 500,000 people have enrolled in the program. Classes are held at 250 locations throughout New Jersey, New York, Pennsylvania, and Florida.

First visits cost six dollars; the remaining sessions in the sixteen-week program are two dollars and fifty cents each.

"His belly was upblown with luxury,
And eke with fatness swollen were his eyne."
—Edmund Spenser, *The Faerie Queene*

BETTER LIVING
155 Bethlehem Pike
Philadelphia, Pennsylvania 19118
Phone: (215) CH2-6930

Better Living programs (including Right Weigh, a weight-reduction program) are all located in and around Philadelphia and operate under the aegis of the Seventh-Day Adventist Church.

The Right Weigh program uses films, lectures, group dynamics, demonstrations, recipes, individual consultations, fitness testing, psychological and medical lectures, and food demonstrations.

The charge is thirty dollars, which includes a control booklet, printed materials, breakfast every day, and entrée samples.

Better Living also offers a course that includes six different classes on cooking and nutrition. You can learn about protein foods, Chinese cooking, vegetarian menus, and foods for maximum health. There are also discussions on overweight, low-calorie and low-cholesterol diets, dieting for all age groups, and facts about fats, vitamins, and minerals, and how to avoid a heart attack. The total cost is ten dollars.

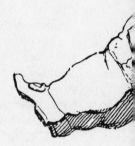

ROBERT SCHACHTER AND
ASSOCIATES
1166 Beacon Street
Brookline, Massachusetts 02146
Phone: (617) 738-0810

Mr. Schachter says that his Method of Eating is *not a diet,* rather it is a training program to allow folks to change their eating patterns. And it's based on psychological principles. This method says there are two types of eating: hunger-based eating and nervous eating.

The training involves exercises which help you distinguish between these two kinds of eating, information on what foods your body needs, a re-education in how to chew your food properly, etc.

The course consists of six weekly group sessions. Follow-up meetings are also available.

Currently the only clinic is at the address above, but within a year there are offices planned for New York and Los Angeles.

The cost of the course is about $100.

WEIGHT COUNSELLING SERVICES
424 Newtonville Avenue
Newtonville, Massachusetts 02160
Phone: (617) 965-4695

The following are the services provided to help you lose weight:

1. Weight Counselling specializes in the unsuccessful dieter on an individual basis.
2. Each person is seen initially for a private diet consultation and a personalized diet plan is worked out. Following this, other sessions are scheduled to check progress and make changes in the diet plan.
3. There is also a Mini-Diet Course to get people going.
4. Also used are behavioral and educational methods.
5. There are also groups for people who have lost weight with individual counseling and can benefit from the success of others.
6. An up-to-date medical report is required.
7. The staff consists of experienced registered nurses and clinical social workers.

"Just keep this motto in front of you:
The feeling of hunger is indispensable to a successful diet."

—Arlene Dahl

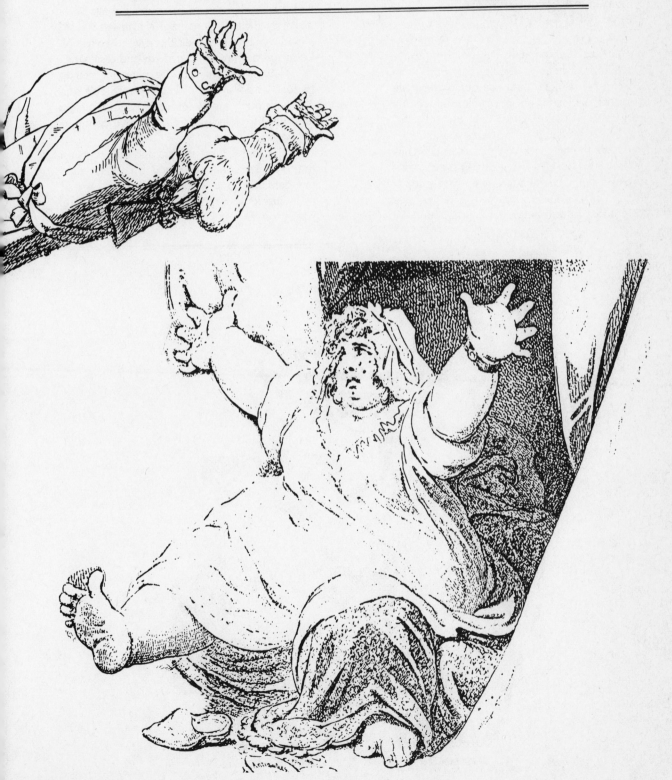

The Midwest

WEIGHT LOSERS INTERNATIONAL
5500 West Capitol Drive
Milwaukee, Wisconsin 53216
Phone: (414) 444-9100

Weight Losers International is a diet group located in 100 cities in eight states. Started in 1968 in Milwaukee, they use our old-favorite diet, the Prudent Diet by Dr. Norman Jolliffe from the New York City Health Department. So you know the diet is nutritionally sound.

Each member of a Weight Losers class has at least ten pounds to lose during the sixteen-week program. Many have much bigger goals. According to Weight Losers: "The average weight loss in that period of time is about 40 pounds." Each class is conducted by a certified instructor who has completed an eight-hour training program.

After reaching goal weight the weight-loser may participate in a free lifetime maintenance program. What Weight Losers tries to teach is not a diet but a new pattern of eating habits.

There is a word that Weight Losers uses that I haven't seen much of in the world of weight reduction—that magical four-letter word *love*. Love is part of their three-word basic philosophy—along with *selectivity* and *discipline*.

Being a romantic I quote you what they try to teach about love: "The love of self and others through a new understanding of weight and weight-related problems." Love conquers all, yes sir.

The cost is three dollars and fifty cents for the initial registration fee and two dollars and fifty cents for each weekly meeting.

Check your phone book for the group nearest you.

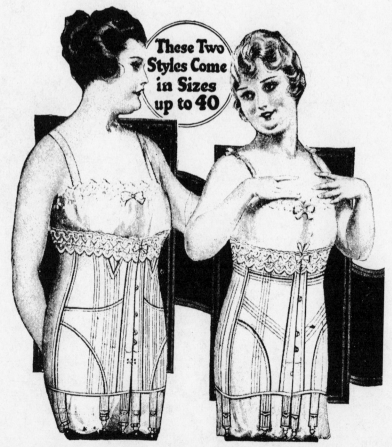

These Two Styles Come in Sizes up to 40

For Stout Figures.   For Short, Stout Figures.

The West

TOTAL IMAGE WORKSHOP
"The People's Centers"
National Busibody Services, Inc.
6343 S. Eastern Avenue, Suite B
Bell Gardens, California 90201
Phone: (213) 771-9666

The Total Image Workshop offers an eight-week course concerned primarily with overweight, and with other related topics such as self-hypnosis and sexuality. The cost is five dollars per session; the course is limited to small groups. Here's a brief rundown on what's cooking at each session.

Session 1: I Am a Person
  experiencing self-discovery
  slender food sampling
Session 2: Alternatives and Attitudes
  exploring new insights in weight control
  slender food sampling
Session 3: Psychological Aspects of Overeating
  lecture, film, and discussion
  slender food sampling
Session 4: Self-Confidence Through Body Image
  achieving your desired total image
  slender food sampling
Session 5: Self-Hypnosis and the Total Image
  learning that you are what you think
Session 6: Exotic Slender Cooking
  a gourmet experience of delicious, economical, and easy-to-prepare foods
  a sip-and-nibble workshop
Session 7: Assertiveness Training
  learning to express your positive self
Session 8: The Art of Sexual Intimacy
  an evening of emerging sensory awareness toward romantic relationships

Each of the sessions is headed by trained consultants. The professionals and paraprofessionals who run the program include a marriage counselor, family counselor, certified consultant in human sexuality, college professor, certified master hypnotist, professional beauty consultant, and licensed psychologist.

It looks to me as if they're trying to change the total you. And if the "total you" is smaller at the end, the fee is certainly low.

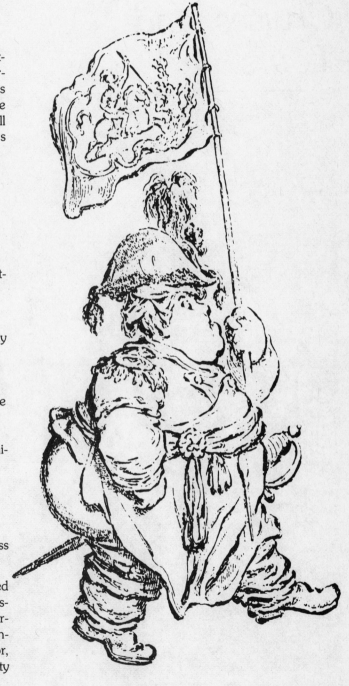

Diet Resorts,
Health Farms,
Camps,
Cruises, and
Tours

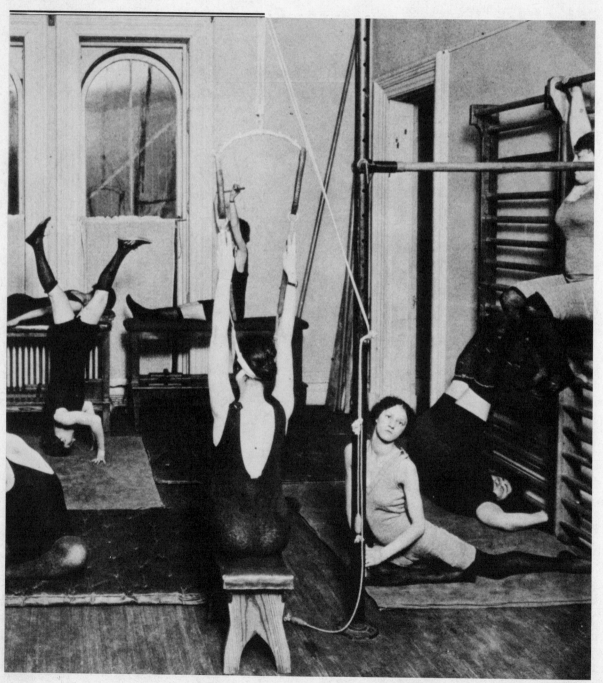

Many folks have to be whisked away to a diet never-never land in order to lose weight. Going away exclusively to lose weight and get in shape has become a very popular and successful way to concentrate on putting the old bod back in its original form.

It's obvious you are there for only one reason. No work, diversions, or pressures to make you overeat. Just diet, exercise, relaxation, and massage until you're a new you. It's like a vacation, except you don't get to eat much.

I have yet to meet anyone who went away to one of these glamorous fat farms and didn't think it was a terrific way to lose weight and inches.

Being a hot diet item, these places can cost from a few hundred dollars to way over a thousand dollars, plus gratuities.

Some are coed, too. Who knows, your social life might pick up. You could get married in the sauna bath.

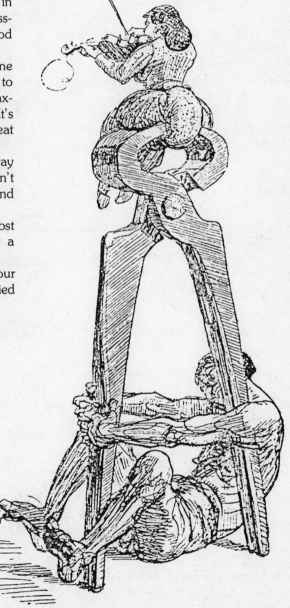

Pinching Cure

Kneippkur

If you think that the closest you'll get to La Costa or The Greenhouse is a quick run through the pages of this book, get a little more detail with

THE GLAMOUR SPAS by Kitty Kelly
$1.50   Paperback   251 pages
Pocket Books

This is one big, juicy, gossipy "tour de fat" through all the places where the rich and famous take it off.

Kitty Kelly spent a week at each resort. She followed the diets, participated in all the programs, talked to the guests, and did the exercises, and she swears she tells the "whole truth within the limits of libel and literary license."

Ms. Kelly covers the whole price range of spas from $185-a-week austerity all the way up to $3000-a-week chicness. She puts them in categories like "status and luxury, swingers and seaside spas for old folks."

But why spas? As Kitty Kelly points out, "Any woman who has ever signed herself into the velvet confines of a fat farm will admit that she could probably do the same job herself without going to a spa. Despite the elegance, she is still eating like a pygmy and sweating like a porpoise. That, as we all know is the only way to become beautifully slim and it's something anyone can do at home. But most of us won't do it ourselves. We want someone to do it for us, or at least make us feel better while doing it." And why not, if you can afford the money and the time.

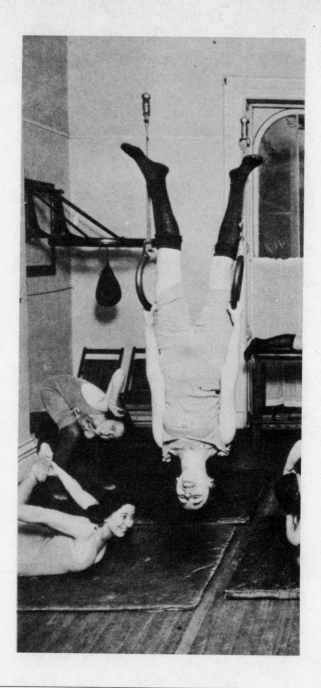

"The pound of flesh which I demand of him Is dearly bought."

ACT IV, SCENE I
The Merchant of Venice

146

The East

CAMELOT CENTERS, INC.
949 Northfield Road
Woodmere, New York 11598
Phone: (516) 374-0785

Location of camps:
Camelot at Union College, Schenectady, New York 12308
Camelot at Gordon College, Wenham, Massachusetts 01984
Camelot at University of North Carolina, Wilmington, North Carolina 28401
Camelot at Whittier College, Whittier, California 90608

Camelot is a weight-reducing camp for women. The camp is for two age groups: teenagers from thirteen to seventeen and young adults from eighteen to thirty-five. According to the brochure, the "average weight loss is 30 pounds."

One of the unique features of Camelot is that the nutrition program was devised and is monitored by Morton B. Glenn, M.D., medical adviser to The Diet Workshop (see page 131 above) and a well-known New York physician specializing in nutritionally correct weight loss. In addition, each campus has a certified registered nutritionist. According to Dr. Glenn: "These diets are designed not only to allow a youngster to lose weight successfully, but to learn the eating basis by which this weight can be kept off permanently." The camps do not use pills, medications, gimmicks, or crash or fad diets.

Camelot's camp sessions run approximately six weeks and cost from $1200 to $1400, depending on the camp.

Also, according to the brochure, "Internal Revenue Service has indicated that the camp fees may be deductible under proper circumstances. Confer with your accountant and refer to Ruling 55-261 under heading of MEDICAL DEDUCTIONS FOR HEALTH INSTITUTES' FEES."

Maybe Uncle Sam can pay for the weight reduction. No wonder he's skinny.

PAWLING HEALTH MANOR
Robert R. Gross, Director
Box 401, Hyde Park, New York 12538
Phone: (914) 889-4141

The Pawling Health Manor is a year-round "retreat" where "controlled regimens of fasting, exercise and natural nutrition are used."

The gang at Pawling guarantee that you will "lose up to 10 to 20 pounds in the first week." That's what I said. They guarantee that much weight loss.

There is no medical advice given at Pawling. The brochure suggests that "you consult with your physician prior to coming to Pawling Health Manor." And smoking is not permitted at any time.

The first few days of fasting you relax, read, and attend lectures on nutrition and the

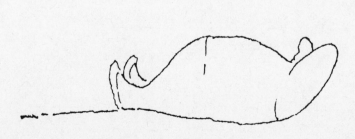

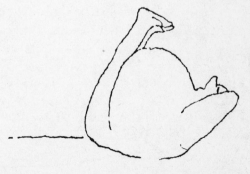

psychology of eating. You drink only well water. The last few days you can eat fruits and vegetables and do a little physical activity in the gym. Pawling Health Manor suggests that you bring a radio, personal stationery, and plenty of reading material.

The rates are reasonable and start at $147 per week. They may not give you much to eat, but that "well water" could very well be the Fountain of Youth.

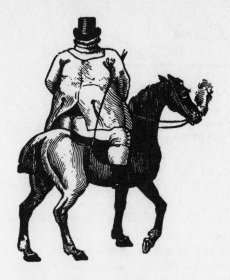

NEW AGE HEALTH FARM
Route 55
Neversink, New York 12765
Phone: (914) 985-7420

Elza and Graeme Graydon, the owners of New Age Health Farm, give a straightforward philosophy of their resort. People have to listen to their bodies. If they do this, their bodies will go in the right direction.

This is primarily a fasting resort, but you can choose to eat if you want to. About seventy percent of the guests fast. The faster drinks or eats nothing but fruit juices, vegetable juices, and herbal teas. A pound a day is the average weight loss over a thirty-day period, provided you don't cheat. According to Ms. Graydon, "Fasting takes away the curtain from the subconscious and brings out feelings that have been squashed by food—anger, jealousy, despair and grief."

She also gives classes in nutrition, yoga, and meditation. You can swim, hike, and do calisthenics, too. The purpose of New Age is health rather than beauty.

The Farm is seventy miles from New York City and has a capacity of seventy guests. There is a wide range of rates, so write them directly, oh hungry one.

CLOVER LODGE, LTD.
Hunter, New York, in Greene County
**   12442**
Phone: (518) 263-9981

Clover Lodge is a camp exclusively for overweight girls from eight to twenty years old. The camp offers a wide variety of activities both athletic and cultural.

A dietician plans the menus, prepares the meals and supervises the kitchen staff. There is no medication of any kind used in the weight reduction program. Consideration is also given to individual dietary needs.

According to the pictures in the brochure, Clover Lodge has plenty for the young ladies to do. There's a big swimming pool, tennis, arts and crafts, slimnastics, and all sorts of things.

Clover Lodge, run by Mrs. William Fershtman, is the second oldest camp for overweight girls.

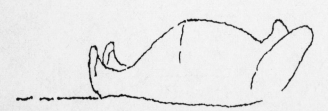

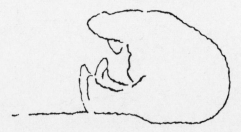

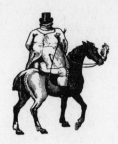

THE ORIGINAL ENGLEWOOD CLIFFS MILK FARM
619 Palisade Avenue
Englewood Cliffs, New Jersey 07632
Phone: (201) 568-5502

This is a milk farm for women only. You ladies can dine on a high-protein or liquid diet. There's a plenty to do with massages, sauna, steam treatment, outdoor swimming pool, and all sorts of activities to make you youthful and invigorated. You will come home beautiful, rested, relaxed, and rejuvenated. I wonder, if I slip on a wig . . .

CAMP STANLEY
Hurleyville, New York 12747
Phone: (914) 434-7780
(516) 484-4240

Camp Stanley is a nonmedical slim-down camp for girls. The Camp is divided into six small camps by age. The "camps within a camp" group the girls with only a year's difference in age.

According to the brochure, the average weight loss is twenty to forty-five pounds. There's also a follow-up program with Mrs. Gussie Mason, Camp Director, that lasts the rest of the year. All the meals are supervised by a nutritionist.

The young women get plenty of exercise with twenty tennis courts, a nine-hole par 3 golf course, and a heated swimming pool.

The camp season starts about July 1 and lasts eight weeks. The total cost is $1730 with no extra charges except for horseback riding, which is optional.

Also the brochure says, "Internal Revenue Service has indicated that the camp fees may be deductible under proper circumstances. Confer with your accountant and refer to Ruling 55-261 under heading of MEDICAL DEDUCTIONS FOR HEALTH INSTITUTES' FEES."

LIDO SPA HOTEL
Belle Island
Venetian Causeway
Miami Beach, Florida 33139
Phone: (800) 327-8363

Suppose you could go to a spa that guarantees weight loss and offers a complete on-arrival medical checkup, individually tailored programs for weight control, a dietician who sees you at every meal, special diets (salt-free, sugar-free, fat-free, bland), and golf and tennis five minutes away? It's located in Miami Beach, Florida, and costs twenty-seven to sixty-three dollars a day, depending on how many are in a room and on the season.

That's the Lido Spa.

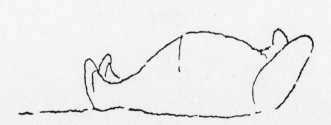

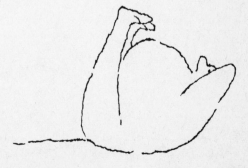

DIETARY BEHAVIORAL CENTER
P.O. Box 013660, Flagler Station
Miami, Florida 33101
Phone: (305) 374-6100 or (800) 327-7400

Judging by the brochure, letter, and publicity they've sent me, this has to be one of the most comprehensive weight-reducing programs. I'll give you a very brief point-by-point description of the program.

1. The program is a four-week weight-reduction plan that is done while you are a resident at the Everglades Hotel in Miami, Florida.
2. The Center is part of the University of Miami School of Medicine. When you arrive you are given a thorough physical examination at the University of Miami School of Medicine.
3. You are also checked daily by a member of the medical staff of the University of Miami Medical School.
4. The Dietary Behavioral Center will approach your obesity from many angles. You will be given a diet of about 900 calories a day. There will be exercises prescribed especially for you by cardiologists. You will learn about nutrition, cooking, and shopping. The big push, and the key to staying on the diet and keeping the weight off, is behavioral modification. You will be flooded with lectures and group sessions to give you a new set of eating habits.
5. Now, dear reader, there are some special requirements—mainly time and money. The course takes four weeks in residence. But's it's in Miami, so what could be bad? As for the cost, the most inexpensive accommodations are $2240 when you share

a room. The prices go up from there. So it's not cheap. Now for the good news. If you are eligible, Medicare and other health insurers will pay a portion of the cost. And if it works, it could be the biggest bargain of your life.

My advice is to write or call the Center and get all the poop in greater detail. The program looks terrific to me, but check it out for yourself.

RENAISSANCE REVITALIZATION CENTER
P.O. Box N4854
Cable Beach, Nassau, Bahamas
Phone: (809) 32-78441-2

The philosophy of Renaissance is to treat the total individual. More than a diet spa, Renaissance is a health center. Under the co-direction of Dr. Ivan Popov and Dr. Elliott Goldwag, the Center is devoted to reestablishing body health and harmony.

Upon entering, an individual's present health and past medical history are evaluated. This is followed by a lengthy discussion to determine current stress condition; then the Center's ten-day program to place the individual back in balance begins.

According to Doctors Popov and Goldwag, the problem of losing weight is a complicated one not solved by the latest fad diet or crash program.

Renaissance recommends to each client an individual diet determined by their medical staff. Clients are also offered general nutritional advice about the kinds of food they should eat for best performance, and the kinds of food they should avoid (such as white refined sugar, white flour, and those foods containing large

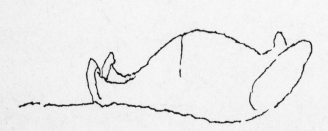
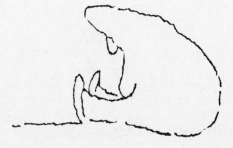

amounts of chemical preservatives) because of their detrimental effects.

Renaissance stresses eating properly balanced proportions of proteins, carbohydrates, and fats. And they believe in the importance of introducing "live" foods into the diet. According to their literature on what they call "embryotherapy," the embryos from their specially incubated chicken eggs can be useful as stimulants and revitalizing agents.

While some weight loss usually does occur during the ten-day program, Renaissance discourages sudden massive changes; they use a gradual stepdown, plateau procedure which enables the body to readjust itself at different states of equilibrium as the person reduces.

Folks who go to Renaissance usually stay at the hotels on Cable Beach next to the Center. They provide all the resort hotel facilities.

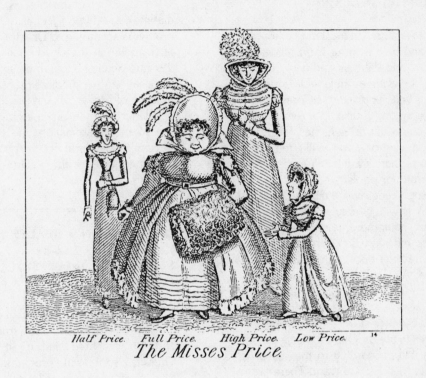

Half Price.   Full Price.   High Price.   Low Price.   14
The Misses Price.

"O, that this too too solid flesh would melt . . ."

ACT I, SCENE 2
Hamlet

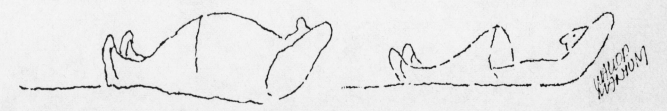

Midwest and Southwest

OLYMPIA PRINCESS RESORT
P.O. Box 208, Dept. GP
Oconomowoc, Wisconsin 53066
Phone: Toll Free: (800) 558-9573
In Wisconsin: (414) 567-0311

This is a new 318-acre resort located two hours from Chicago and half an hour from Milwaukee. Listen you Arnie Palmers and Jack Nicklauses, there's an eighteen-hole golf course. For you Chris Everts and Jimmy Connorses, you can choose among four indoor and three outdoor tennis courts. If you're Esther Williams or Johnny Weismuller, or if you're like me and need water wings, there's a beachfront as well as indoor and outdoor pools.

To get in top shape, two "Million Dollar" health spas beckon with twenty-seven different kinds of exercise equipment, whirlpools, Grecian showers (sounds very sexy), sauna baths, steam room, ultraviolet booth, and eucalyptus inhalation room. Ah—and there are massages available for men and women by hand or by planetary percussion relaxer (sounds like something from *Star Trek*).

The pictures in the brochure look spectacular. The rates vary, according to the season and the accommodations you want. There are several package deals, such as a Sports Spectacular, a Leisure Package, and a Honeymoon Package. Call them toll-free or write.

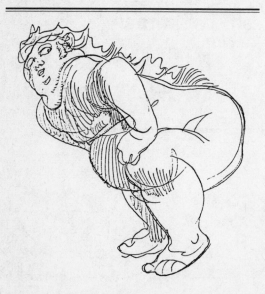

TURNER CLINIC, P.A.
667 South 55th Street
Kansas City, Kansas 66106
Phone: (913) 287-1414
(816) 471-5410

The Turner Clinic, headed by James F. Holleman, Jr., D.O. (Doctor of Osteopathy), is a general or family practice clinic with an emphasis on obesity and cardiovascular diseases.

Obesity, arteriosclerosis, hypertension, diabetes, and hypoglycemia are all diet-related problems according to Dr. Holleman. Because of his belief in the close relationship between diet and health, nutrition plays a major role in his treatment of medical problems and in his practice of preventative medicine.

Dr. Holleman is a member of the American Medical Association, the Kansas Medical Society, the Natural Foods Associates, and the International Academy of Preventative Medicine.

DR. SHELTON'S HEALTH SCHOOL
Route 10, Box 174-E
San Antonio, Texas 78216
Phone: (512) 497-3613

The Health School offers a diet of unprocessed and unrefined foods: fresh fruits, vegetables, and nuts, prepared without salt or condiments. There is also a fasting program, which requires total abstinence from all foods, although you may drink all the water you want.

There are no drugs used at the school. The Health School offers lectures, literature, question periods, and tape recordings to instruct the health-seeker.

The cost runs from $147 weekly to $189 weekly with a $25 entrance fee for each guest.

The West

FANTASTIC FIGURE
10119 West 37th Place
Wheat Ridge, Colorado 80033
Phone: (303) 424-1079

If you ever wanted to be a thin mummy, this is the place. (The brochure didn't mention thin daddys.) The reducing deal here is that you're wrapped in elastic that has been soaked in a warm saline (salt base) solution. The saline solution, according to Fantastic Figure, is "perfectly harmless and nonallergenic. Every ingredient has been approved by the Food and Drug Administration." Don't take a swig; although it's harmless, it's very bitter. Back to the wrap. After you're wrapped, you slip on a plastic coat, lie down, talk with the other mummys, read, gossip, sleep, or make believe you're Cleopatra drifting down the Nile.

With the Fantastic Body Wrap, the theory is that you eliminate the fat directly under the skin. It also works on getting rid of cellulite. But for "deep fat," you still need a proper diet. There are five diets, but they will give you one only after taking your medical history, eating habits, etc.

Again, according to the brochure, "Anyone can be wrapped except people with a very bad heart, or people with phlebitis (a circulatory condition). If there is any doubt, we ask the lady to check with her doctor about being wrapped snugly."

You women can get wrapped twice a week until you've reached your figure goals. You can even get your face wrapped.

PRICE LIST
Introductory Wrap $20.00
Single Wraps $25.00

Wrap Series	*Regular Price*	*First Visit Discount*
Series of 6 wraps	$135.00	$99.00
Series of 20 wraps	$330.00	$195.00
Face Wraps $7.00 each or 5 face wraps $30.00		

10 wraps $132.00
15 wraps $165.00

"Your means are very slender, and your waste is great. I would it were otherwise; I would my means were greater, and my waist slenderer."
ACT I, SCENE 2
Henry IV, Part II

153

THE GOLDEN DOOR
Box 1567
Escondido, California 92025
Phone: (714) 744-5777

A beautiful rural Japanese setting, diet, exercise, beauty treatments, small talk with the big shots such as Barbra Streisand, breakfast in bed, and an average weight loss of five pounds a week are all yours at The Golden Door spa.

Diets are geared to individual guests with an average day's eating pegged at 800 calories. As the founder, Deborah Mazzanti, says, "A high vitality life depends on high vitality food." The food is low-calorie, low-cholesterol, and natural. The chef even teaches you the secrets of how to make low-calorie foods delicious. When you go home, The Golden Door tells you to go back on your specific diet one week a month.

At a typical dinner, you may dine on stuffed mushrooms, mixed salad with vinaigrette dressing, veal escalope Florentine, baby carrots and snow peas macedoine, and chocolate mousse. Sounds wonderful as long as someone else is doing the cooking.

For us guys, there are eight different men's weeks scattered throughout the year so we can get slim and handsome too. The cost is $1250 per week plus 15-percent gratuity. There are also special mother-daughter weeks, father-son weeks, and couple weeks.

LA COSTA HOTEL & SPA
Rancho La Costa
Carlsbad, California 92008
Phone: (714) 438-9111

Beautiful people are all over the place. From the pictures, I can't figure out whether they were gorgeous before they got there or whether luxurious La Costa made them over. Probably a combination of both.

Anyone who's ever heard of any spa has heard of La Costa in southern California. How's the weather? Summer average: seventy-four degrees. Winter average: sixty-eight degrees. Perfect.

You can go on two plans, the European plan (not for dieters, so we won't discuss it further) or the Spa plan. There are two Spas, one for women and one for men. On the Spa plan you will meet the medical director and dietician. The result will be a personal program designed to meet your individual objectives. You can relax, reshape, revitalize.

There's a championship golf course, twenty-five tennis courts, and classes in just about everything. And it's only five minutes from the Pacific Ocean, and forty-five minutes from Disneyland.

There are five restaurants and you can diet on such yummies as rock lobster tails and low-calorie chocolate mousse.

Now you may ask, how much? Double, on the complete Spa Plan, $180 per day; single, on complete Spa Plan, $120 per day. On both plans you must add 15-percent service charge and 6-percent tax.

"When you sit down to eat with a ruler
Observe carefully what is before you;
And put a knife to your throat
If you are a man given to appetite.
Do not desire his delicacies,
For they are deceptive food.

Proverbs 23:1-3

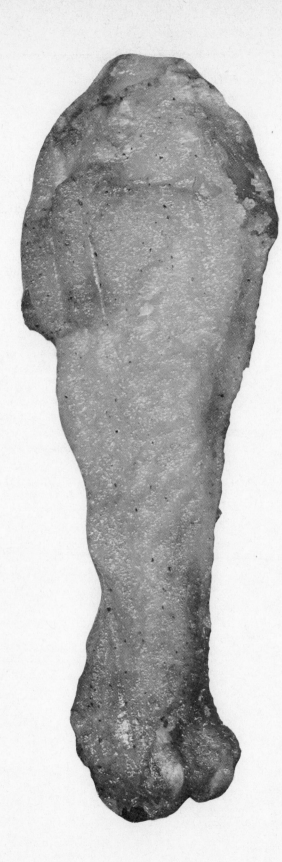

RANCHO LA PUERTA
Tecate, Baja California, Mexico
Tecate, California 92080
Phone: (714) 478-5400

Pals who have gone to Rancho La Puerta think it's the greatest thing since sliced bread. (The ranch is famous, by the way, for its whole grain bread.)

Located thirty miles southeast of San Diego, it's only a three-hour drive from smoggy Los Angeles to 150 fogless, smogless acres of rolling hills.

Rancho La Puerta was founded in 1940 by Ms. Deborah Mazzanti, who also founded The Golden Door Spa.

There's room for about 100 guests and it's coed. The Ranch is the largest spa in this hemisphere totally dedicated to a full-time fitness program. You can choose from tennis courts, putting green, nine gyms (three of them outdoors), three swimming pools, volleyball court, and whirlpool-jet therapy pool.

La Puerta is known for its 1000-calorie vegetarian slimming diet (also low-sodium and low-cholesterol) built around natural foods. These are well-chosen calories that will not leave you hungry or lacking in energy.

Okay, how much? Not much, really.

	For Two—Each	For One
Las Haciendas (small homes)	$65.00	Unavailable
Las Rancheras	$55.00	$70.00
Las Cabanas (studios)	$45.00	$60.00
Las Casitas	$40.00	$50.00

These rates are effective December 1, 1976.

If you're even mildly interested, write for their literature. The brochures are terrific.

THE MURRIETA
Murrieta Hot Springs, California
Phone: (714) 677-5611

The Murrieta is a resort hotel, country club, and spa designed to invigorate, relax, and make that old bod feel like new.

There are all sorts of rubs and baths, but the big one is the Tule Root Mud Baths. Personally, I'd rather bathe in whipped cream. But the Mud Baths are supposed to promote relaxation and renewed vitality.

Each guest has a private suite. There are tennis courts, an eighteen-hole championship golf course, a swimming pool, horseback riding, and plenty of social activities. That's for me. More important, there is a Diet Dining Room.

The cost of "The Terrific Toner" (three days) is $285. The cost of "The Fabulous Condition" (one week) is $665.

They advise you to get your doctor's approval before your visit or before starting any of the programs.

SID STOLLER'S
KIOWA LODGE
31750 Riverside Drive
Elsinore, California 92330
Phone: (714) 674-9977

Kiowa Lodge has finally given in. After twenty-three years of catering to women only, for the first time they're now letting men in to lose weight. Hurrah for men's liberation.

This is a weight-control and rest resort based on your individual caloric needs. You may participate in such activities as yoga, dance exercise, facial exercise, pool exercises, daily hikes, mat exercise classes, and calisthenics.

Besides the three meals daily, they also serve early-bird coffee, hot lemon-water wake-up, midmorning and midafternoon juices, and late evening snacks. Kiowa will follow your doctor's special instructions and diets.

The emphasis here is on casual relaxed comfort, so leave your diamonds, furs, and tuxedo at home. Rates start at $29 per day in a double room.

FIVE

PROFESSIONAL HELP

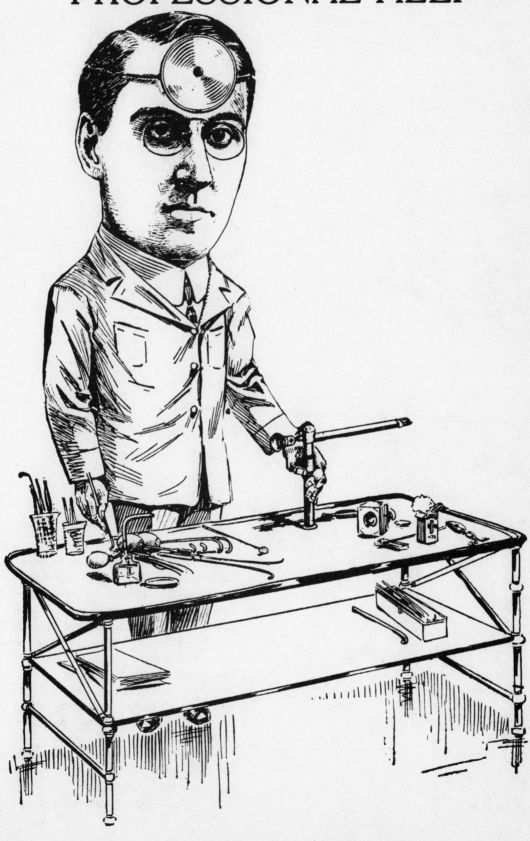

DIET
DOCTORS

Doctors cannot advertise—not yet, anyway. If you want a physician specializing in obesity, ask your family doctor, write the American Society of Bariatric Physicians (see address, page 159), or see what you can find out by word of mouth.

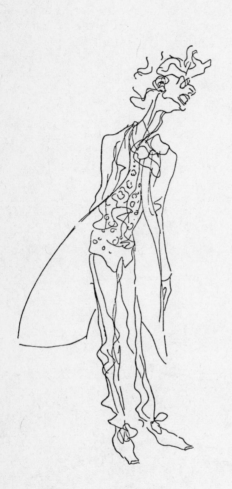

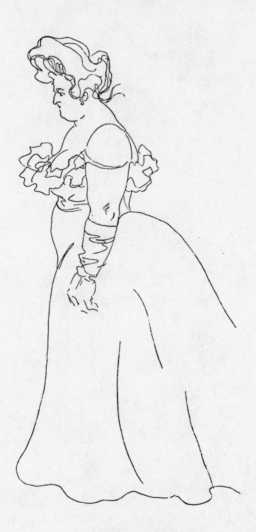

I went to one diet doctor in my life. This was in Kansas City, when I was about sixteen years old. It was like being on a Chevrolet assembly line. You walked in; he took your blood pressure, handed you a mimeographed sheet on what to eat and what not to eat, weighed you, handed you a little bag of pills, shook your hand, smiled, and said good-bye. That was the last time you saw the good doctor. You were supposed to come back every week to be weighed and get your new bag of pills. Of course the pills were Dexedrine—"uppers." He charged you ten bucks for the weigh-in and the pills. After being high for three days and giggling a lot, I flushed those little honeys.

What I'm trying to say is: be very careful.

AMERICAN SOCIETY OF BARIATRIC PHYSICIANS
333 West Hampden Avenue
Englewood, Colorado 80110
Phone: (303) 761-2198

The American Society of Bariatric Physicians is a group of M.D.'s and D.O.'s specializing in obesity and weight control.

The Society has 550 members throughout the United States and Canada, and one each in Mexico and Greece.

The Society also provides a referral service for those interested in finding a bariatrician to help with their overweight problems.

There you are. You can write the Society and find a doctor devoting full time or at least part time to overweight and weight control. There are members in all parts of the country.

WEIGHT CONTROL DYNAMICS
Stanley H. Title, M.D., P.C.
171 West 57th Street
New York, New York 10019
Phone: (212) LT1-9532

Dr. Title has devoted his medical practice exclusively to the treatment of overweight.

His office, which includes on its staff a dietary–behavior modification advisor, treats the individual according to his own specific needs, which are determined by a physical examination and laboratory (and other) tests.

According to Dr. Title, "The programs include injectible methods, low carbohydrate diets, balanced diets, protein sparing and other short term fasts—along with proper and safe medication as indicated and a program to assist in changing the individual's eating and living patterns."

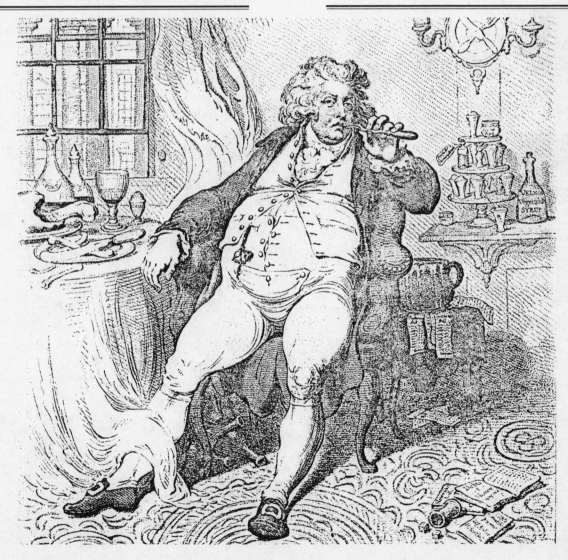

ALEXANDER MATOS, D.O.
176 East 75th Street
New York, New York
Phone: (212) 763-7614

Dr. Matos is a licensed New York State chiropractor and is a past president of the American Hypnotist Association.

The guiding principle in his weight-reduction program is called Vicarious Sexual Motivative Factor. As he says, "Simply stated, the V.S.M. Factor measures the pleasure that one obtains from being sexually attractive to the opposite sex."

In order to lose weight, we must up our V.S.M. Factor. Once we're motivated, we trade the satisfaction that food gives us to the bigger pleasure of being thin and good-looking.

Dr. Matos tells us, "You and you alone make the decision to eat or not to eat. Properly motivate yourself and you can be thin."

I've never been hypnotized. And I don't know if being sexually attractive was my only motivation for losing 170 pounds. But I'm sure that I was the horniest 320-pound man west of the Mississippi. As for you, dear reader, what can I tell you about the strength of the sex drive that you don't already know?

THE HUMAN DEVELOPMENT CENTER
Marvin S. Goldstein, Ph.D.
2050 Peachtree Industrial Court
Suite 114-E
Chamblee, Georgia 30341
Phone: (404) 455-0400

The Human Development Center is a psychological center that specializes in using hypnosis to help people lose weight.

The consultation fee is forty dollars; most sessions are about the same price.

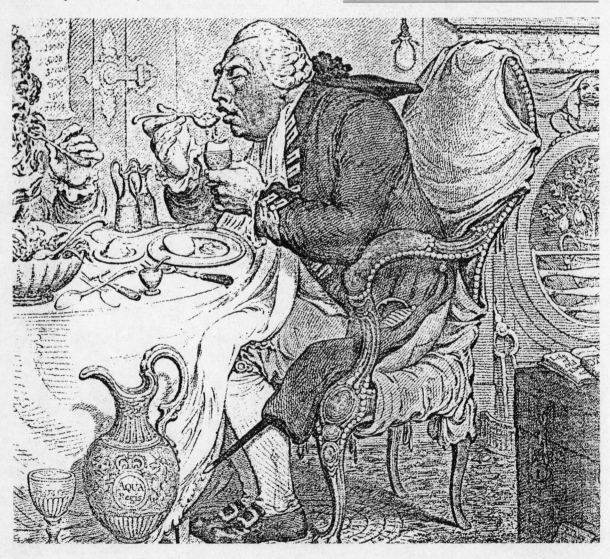

ALFRED W. FERRISS, M.D.
Medical Weight Reduction
516 Sutter Street
San Francisco, California 94102
Phone: (415) 433-1515

This doctor offers a twenty-one-day program. The primary medication used is HCG, or Human Chorionic Gonadotropin—a protein hormone (recovered from human urine and placentas) which has become popular in many diet programs. Other oral medications are also used when needed.

The diet is limited to 500 calories or less per day. According to the brochure there are permissible and forbidden foods:

1. "Black Hats (absolutely forbidden)"—such things as alcohol, sugar, starches, and marijuana (I guess you can't get high and get low in the weight department).
2. "Grey Hats (probably bad, use with caution)"—Milk and dairy products of all kinds, eggs, almost all red meats, dark poultry, most fish and salt.
3. "White Hats (permitted and encouraged)"—
   Vegetables: such crunchies as asparagus, carrots, and celery.
   Seasonings and spices: vinegar, lemon, oregano, etc.
   Beverages: no less than ten eight-ounce volumes . . . black coffee, tea, and artificially sweetened soft drinks.
   Fruits: apples, oranges, etc., but "shun fruit juices."
   Protein: Twice per week—200 calories each time—boiled chicken, lobster, veal, etc.

The brochure also mentions a Ten-Day Cleansing Diet:

Three days: four to six apples and two to three quarts of water only.
Seven days: 500 calories of vegetables only and three to six quarts of fluid—no less than two and a half quarts of water.

MARTIN SCHIFF, M.D.
12900 Venice Boulevard
Los Angeles, California

Dr. Schiff has treated thousands of overweight men and women since 1951. He has also written a book called *Doctor Schiff's Miracle Weight-Loss Guide,* 224 pages, Hardbound, $7.95, Parker Publishing Co.

Very briefly I'll give you some of the Good Doctor's diet tips.

1. Eat more often: Instead of three meals a day eat five or six times a day, but gradually decrease the daily amount of food.
2. Doctor Shiff says, "This is an eating program, not a noneating program! You can be full and still lose weight. Eat high-protein, low-fat, low-carbohydrate foods for weight loss and good nutrition."
3. Eat slowly. Learn to enjoy each bite. "Go into slow motion at the table."
4. You have to tell the difference between hunger and appetite. "Appetite is psychological, emotional. People turn to food instead of learning to cope with their feelings and emotions. Hunger is a normal, physical response. Eat only when you're hungry. Feed your hunger, not your appetite."
5. Watch out for situations that lead to false hunger or appetite, such as parties, watching TV, boredom, and rewarding yourself after a hard day.
6. List things you can do to avoid an eating crisis, such as talking to a friend, meditating, taking a shower, riding your bike, singing, etc.
7. Deal with your emotions and feelings. Give yourself a self-evaluation through writing and meditating.
8. Work toward improving your self-image. All you have to do is take responsibility for your life. Self-love is very important.
9. Develop an exercise program for yourself which will get you in shape physically and help you emotionally too.

These all seem like sound principles, but I personally dislike the use of the word "miracle," in the book title. Anyone who's ever been on a diet for over fifteen minutes knows there's no such thing. The only miracle in dieting for me is how I got by a McDonalds without running in for a double order of French fries.

KATHY KING ASSOCIATES
Kathy King, R.D., dietician
8403 Bryant
Westminster, Colorado 80030
Phone: (303) 427-3035

3201 East 2nd
Cherry Creek, Colorado
Phone: (303) 322-4212

There's one sure thing about dieting and nutrition, you never know all the answers. New discoveries and help about food are always just around the corner. I sometimes think it would be good to marry a dietician or nutritionist and we could sit around and talk about food all the time. On the other hand, maybe it's not such a good idea. I'd probably get so hungry I'd get fat again.

Here's what dietician Kathy King says about her program:

"Patients are referred to me by their physicians for all medical diets. Weight control is our specialty, and we have had very good luck with people losing weight, and then keeping it off afterward. For all diets, we urge people to use normal foods whenever possible and try to avoid the more expensive 'dietetic' products. Exercise is also stressed for persons who can handle it. At present all consultation is individual, but we have plans to begin again with group sessions within the year.

"We charge $15-$20 for the initial visit of approximately one hour, and $5 for revisits."

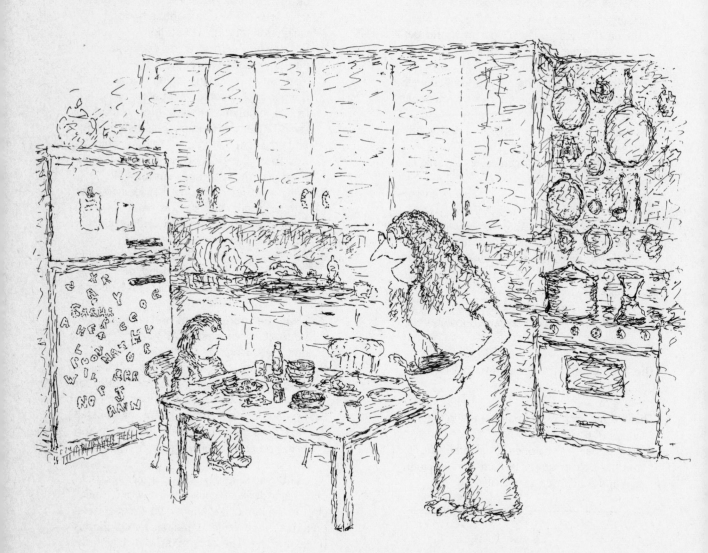

"No more carbohydrates until you finish your protein."

Obesity Clinics

Obesity clinics are usually for the very obese—people who weigh 400, 500, or 600 pounds. Most clinics are associated with hospitals or universities that are doing obesity research.

If you're interested in a specific clinic, call it and find out exactly what its requirements are for becoming a patient.

If you don't know of any clinics in your area, call your local hospital for information. There may be an outpatient obesity clinic in your town or nearby. You'd be surprised at the information you can get by making a couple of calls.

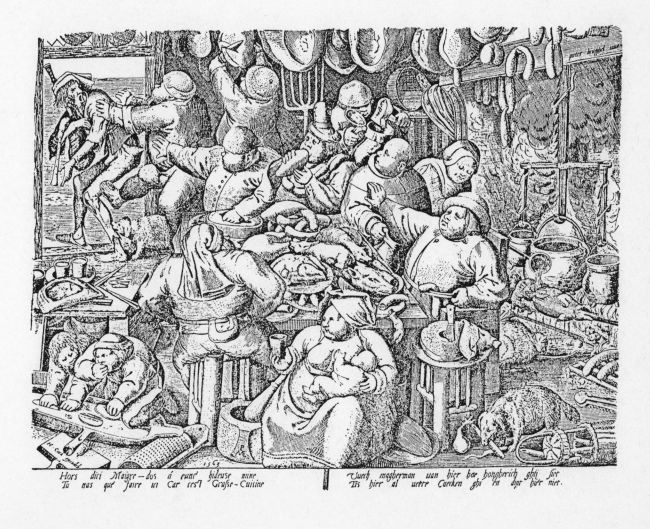

Hors dici Maigre—dos á eunt hideuse mine
Tu nas que faire ui Car cest Graſſe-Cuisine

Vuech magherman uan hier bae horghrich ghij ſiet
Tis hier al uette Cuecken ghi ên duer hie'r niet.

WALTER KEMPNER FOUNDATION, INC.
Box 3099, Duke University Medical Center
Durham, North Carolina 27710
Phone: (919) 684-8111

The Rice Diet was developed in the late 1930s and early 1940s at the Duke University School of Medicine by Dr. Walter Kempner. The diet was originally for people with severe kidney disease. Dr. Kempner then adapted the diet for patients with high blood pressure, hardening of the arteries, and diabetes. Recently he adapted the Rice Diet to the treatment of obesity.

The basic diet is cooked rice, either white or brown, fruit, tea, and sugar. According to the *Archives of Internal Medicine*, December 1975, the initial diet is low-calorie, low-salt, low-protein, low-fat, and essentially free of cholesterol.

At least a month after starting, vegetables are added and still later lean poultry or meats are added. The dieter must also take multivitamins every day.

You must live in the Durham area. There are daily checks of your weight and blood pressure plus consultations with physicians or patient counselors.

The Rice Diet is for massive obesity and must be followed under the strict care of a physician. It sounds monotonous as hell, but if you've got a huge overweight problem you might want to consider it. Talk to your doctor and write for information at the above address.

You might take comfort from the fact that a lot of show biz personalities tried it and were successful. You too can join the stars.

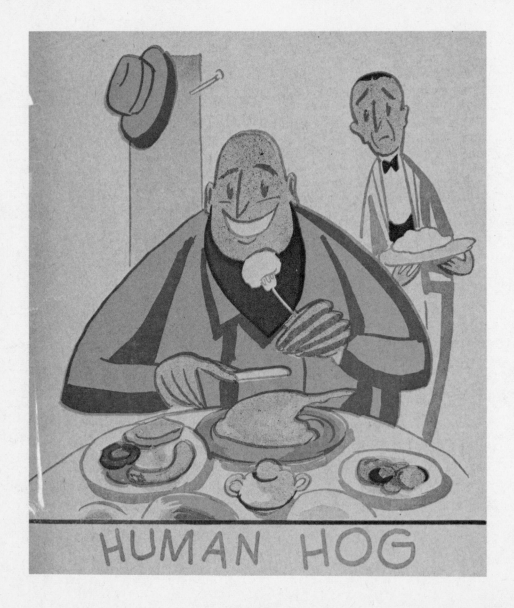

HUMAN HOG

PROFESSIONAL WEIGHT CONTROL, LTD.
11055 Cedar—Suite 216
Cedar Parkway Professional Building
Overland Park, Kansas 66211
Phone: (913) 341-6161

Here's another place which has an HCG program. The following selected quotes from their own brochure will best describe it:

"The treatment is never less than 28 days (25 injections plus 3 additional days of diet alone), regardless of the amount of weight loss required. It takes at least three weeks to regain the normal fat regulating capacity of the appetite control center of the brain. By giving repeated courses 100 or even 200 pounds may be lost without any hardship to the patient. As many courses as are necessary may be given until normal weight is attained.

"The treatment must be closely supervised for optimum results. You will weigh every day, and if there is no loss, an explanation must be found. The average weight loss of one-half to one pound daily is expected. This must occur, or a suitable reason to explain a lack of loss should be found.

"Since each patient is an individual, we design a diet program and HCG injection schedule to suit their special problems and needs."

What is HCG (Human Chorionic Gonadotrophin)? "It's a substance which occurs naturally in a pregnant woman."

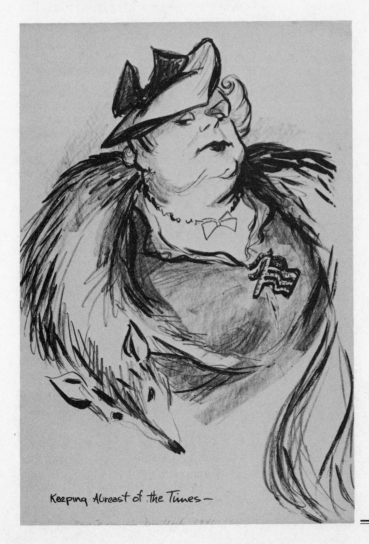

Keeping Abreast of the Times—

When are fat cells formed? According to the director of a children's obesity program at New York's Mount Sinai Hospital, fat cells are formed during three distinct periods: during the last three months before birth, from birth to the age of two years, and during adolescence.

It's not enough that we grow older—we also grow fatter. For the average American, there is a steady gain of one pound a year, every year, after the age of twenty-five.

CORONADO METABOLIC CLINIC
WEIGHT CONTROL
579 Orange Avenue
Coronado, California 92118
Phone: (714) 435-0164

The Coronado Metabolic Clinic offers several diet regimens for you to choose from: the Simeon system of HCG injections (see page 167) plus diet; the Protein Sparing Modified Fast; and other kinds of diet and medication programs.

Which plan is selected for you depends on your degree of obesity, life-style, and various aspects of your physical make-up such as hormonal functions and metabolic levels.

The prospective patient is given a thorough work-up and consultations with the director and medical director before starting any program.

SUNSET MEDICAL CENTER
77 Mark Drive
San Rafael, California 94903
Phone: (415) 664-2248

The underlying philosophy of weight control adopted by the Sunset Medical Center is that learning to control one's habits and under-exercising is the key to success in losing weight and keeping it off.

The habit modification which they teach consists of processes whereby patients learn to foresee and "fore-feel" the negative consequences of eating high-calorie food so vividly they are able to choose to avoid it. Hypnosis may be offered as a way to augment the habit modification process if necessary.

Sunset also has an acupuncture weight-loss program. While a patient is wearing the ear "staple," which is properly termed a "press needle," he or she is also practicing self-administered "habit modification."

At present there are three clinics in the San Francisco Bay area. Call the number above for referral to any clinic.

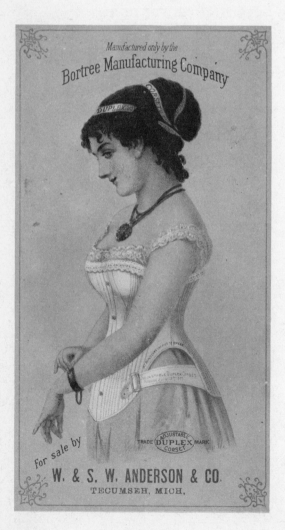

Manufactured only by the
Bortree Manufacturing Company

For sale by
W. & S. W. ANDERSON & CO.
TECUMSEH, MICH.

"I hope that he that looks upon me will take me without weighing."
ACT 1, SCENE 2
Henry IV, Part II

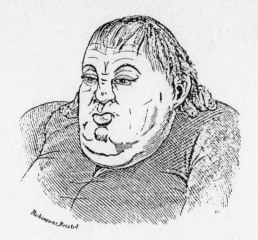

WEIGHT REDUCTION MEDICAL CLINICS, INC.
345 West Portal Avenue, Suite 4A
San Francisco, California 94015
Phone: (415) 665-7034

Another HCG program. Again I quote from the brochure:

The Treatment
"The treatment is never less than 28 days (25 injections plus 3 additional days of diet alone), regardless of the amount of weight loss required."

Daily Injections
"In order to achieve the desired effect on the abnormal adipose tissue fat, HCG must be injected daily for maximum results."

What is HCG?
"It is a substance which occurs naturally in a pregnant woman."

The Diet
"The diet must be followed to the letter! The diet used in conjunction with HCG does not exceed 500 calories per day, and the way these calories are made up is of utmost importance."

The Cost
The cost runs approximately $250, which includes a doctor's physical examination, all laboratory tests, seven weeks of treatments, and three years of maintenance.

MEDICAL DIET SERVICE
1544 S.E. Hawthorne
Portland, Oregon 97214
Phone: (503) 233-5741

MEDICAL DIET SERVICE
1113 Boylston Avenue
Seattle, Washington 98101
Phone: (206) 329-1533

Medical Diet Service is a weight-loss clinic where the emphasis is on learning to eat correctly and on changing eating patterns and habits permanently. Usually you are placed on a diet with a daily intake of 1260 calories, in a wide variety of foods. The daily caloric content includes approximately forty-five grams of carbohydrate, ninety grams of protein, and eighty grams of fat, of which twenty-five percent is polyunsaturated. Food is provided in individually portioned packages which you take home with you: this plan is supposed to help you learn to handle food intake with confidence and a kind of "on-the-job" training.

When you reach normal weight, you are given a maintenance program to follow. Individuals who have reduced to the recommended weight are recalled periodically over a period of two years to assist them in maintaining that weight.

The overweight patient visits a Medical Diet Service office once a week. He or she meets with his counselor privately to discuss his progress, and his weight is charted. At this weekly visit he also receives his food for the next week. However, there are no contractual obligations or fines levied if the weekly schedule is not followed.

Mind Control and Weight Loss

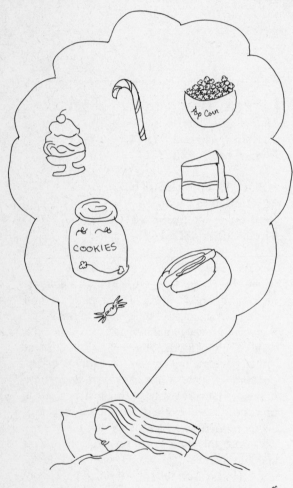

Sasha Chermayeff

As I mosey down the yellow-brick, part-skim-mozzarella-cheese road of life, I am becoming more and more impressed by the effect the mind has in controlling weight.

The newest technique is behavioral modification. That is: become aware of your behavior and your eating habits and then you can learn to change and control them. Behavior modification often requires that you keep a daily recording—when you eat, how you eat, where you eat, with whom you eat, what mood you are in when you eat. This way you will have a blueprint of your exact eating patterns. Correct these and you can lose weight. A great many diet groups and programs are using this technique plus a diet with great success.

Besides behavior modification, we have hypnosis, acupuncture (I'm putting this in the mind category), psychiatry, psychology, mind-benders like EST and Transcendental Meditation, and finally religion. I would approach some of these programs with a grain of salt (nonsodium, of course).

Transcendental Meditation beckoned to me one day. I went to the introductory lectures, laid out 125 smackers, got my mantra, went to the follow-up lectures, and started meditating.

The reason why I started TM was to see if by becoming more relaxed and alert, as they said I would, the hunger pains would ease up. I'm sorry to report they didn't. In fact, they got worse.

Besides getting hungrier, I also got headaches. The TM people said I was straining on my mantra.

Anyway, I gave up meditating after two months. But I'm one of the few TM dropouts. Most TM'ers I've talked to say they never felt better. Maybe I should have used "chocolate" as my mantra. Maybe my expectations were unrealistic. The instructors tell you in the beginning not to expect anything specific from TM. Don't start TM to go on a diet, stop smoking, etc. Just let it happen to you.

With all these mind jobs people are doing now, sometimes I think there are as many mind courses as there are minds. But after seventeen years of dieting, I'm convinced the mind can do more than anything else to help you lose weight and keep it off. Makes sense, because the mind controls your every thought and action. Of course there is physical pain from dieting, but your mind can make it easier and more controllable.

Get your head in shape and your body will follow.

ACUPUNCTURE INFORMATION CENTER OF NEW YORK, INC.
127 East 69th Street, New York, New York 10021
Phone: (212) 535-6400

EAR-ACUPUNCTURE THERAPY FOR WEIGHT LOSS

The Acupuncture Information Center of New York, a nonprofit corporation chartered by the State of New York, says that the Chinese have known for centuries that the ear controls many body functions, especially appetite. As their brochure states: "The most commonly accepted conclusion is that acupuncture blocks certain 'messages' which are sent from the body to the brain." "It must be remembered that no program of assistance to the overweight patient can be successful without the full participation of the patient."

The following is a list of recommended facilities by the Acupuncture Information Center of New York. According to them, each center provides legal and medically supervised acupuncture by Asian experts.

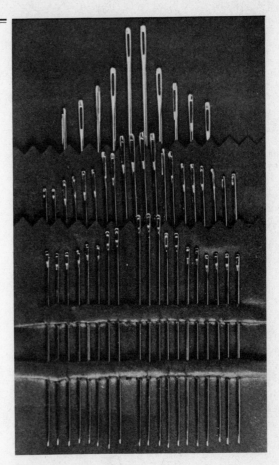

ACUPUNCTURE CENTER OF NEW YORK
426 East 89th Street
New York, New York 10028
Phone: (212) 534-6800

ACUPUNCTURE CENTER OF WASHINGTON
1712 I Street, N.W.
Washington, D.C. 20006
Phone: (202) 298-5911

ACUPUNCTURE CENTER OF BETHESDA
4400 East-West Highway
Bethesda, Maryland 20014
Phone: (301) 652-2829

MASSACHUSETTS ACUPUNCTURE CENTER
1842 Beacon Street
Brookline, Massachusetts 02146
Phone: (617) 734-8070

ACUPUNCTURE CENTER OF SPRINGFIELD
1537 Main Street
Springfield, Massachusetts
Phone: (413) 788-9666

DALLAS ACUPUNCTURE CENTER
6211 W. Northwest Highway, Rm. 523C
Dallas, Texas 75225
Phone: (214) 361-9531

MORPHEUS ENTERPRISES, LTD.
Jerome Walman
425 East 51st Street, Suite 1D
New York, New York 10022
Phone: (212) PL5-4363

Mr. Walman offers hypnosis and meditation for weight reduction and control. He used to be 100 pounds heavier, but he lost weight and kept it off with hypnosis.

All sessions are by appointment only, but for out-of-towners telephone sessions are available.

Prices will be given upon request.

GROUP CONDITIONING ASSOCIATES, INC.
An Affiliate of
New York Institute for Hypnotherapy
One Barstow Road
Great Neck, New York 11021
Phone: (516) 829-5969

The Hypno-Dietetics workshop consists of a total of four hours. During this four-hour period, each participant is taught how to respond effectively to hypnosis and to induce self-hypnosis to change his eating habits.

The program of hypnosis, complemented by self-hypnosis, along with a taped recording, is designed to reinforce suggestions to improve participants' eating patterns and help them lose weight.

There is a charge of sixty-five dollars per person, which includes all services and materials, for the four-hour session.

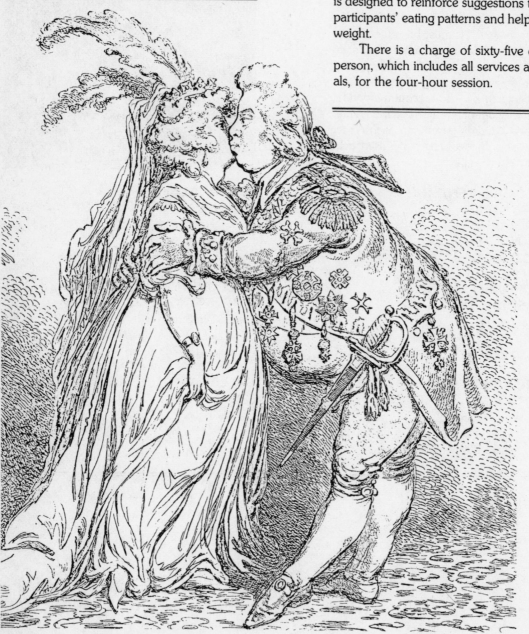

HYPNOLOGY CENTER
Frank Rocco, R.H. (Registered Hypnologist)
9622 Bustleton Avenue
Philadelphia, Pennsylvania 19115
Phone: (215) 671-0569 Appointments Only

Mr. Rocco has developed a plan known as Audio-Therapy. With Audio (or listening)-Therapy he uses a "progressive-relaxation" method where overweight folks are motivated to change their eating habits, use whatever diet they desire and help visualize themselves at the weight they want to be.

A variation on this is the Lose Weight While Sleeping Plan where "a person wishing to lose weight can listen to the record before going to sleep at night, and it helps them stay on any diet which they are trying to follow. This works on the same principle as sleep learning."

The price of the recording or cassette tape is nine dollars and may be purchased through the above address.

WEIGHT & TENSION REDUCERS INC.
6666 Security Boulevard
Baltimore, Maryland 21207
Phone: (301) 944-6060

Weight & Tension Reducers uses hypnosis as one part of a behavior modification program for weight loss. They have both group and private sessions. In the weight-reduction group session the first half hour is spent in discussing nutrition and overeating. The second half is devoted to hypnotizing and relaxation. Each person receives individual suggestions designed for him while the rest of the group sits back in recliners listening to soothing music and suggestions through headphones. Auto-suggestion is taught when the goal weight is reached.

I feel more relaxed just reading this.

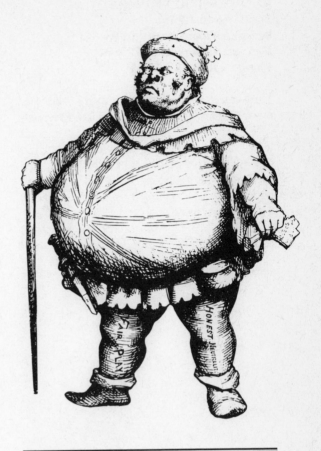

AMERICAN INSTITUTE OF HYPNOTHERAPY COUNSELING CENTER
5918 North Broad Street
Philadelphia, Pennsylvania 19141
Phone: (215) WA 7-0216

According to the people at the American Institute of Hypnotherapy, there is nothing that hypnosis can't straighten out in your mind, including your problem with cherry pie à la mode.

The program is designed individually for each patient. Also included is learning the technique of self-hypnosis so that you can control your weight and keep your desired weight.

AMERICAN CLINIC, INC.
1660 South Albion
Writer's Tower, Suite 520
Denver, Colorado 80222
Phone: (303) 758-4544

The American Clinic offers a form of self-hypnosis for weight control. The training involves weekly visits and the program lasts three to eight weeks. At the end of the training, a tape recording is given the patient to help him keep his weight loss for the rest of his life. If there are any problems after the three to eight weeks, help is given at no charge.

Fees vary with the individual programs, usually twenty-five to thirty dollars per session.

THE NATIONAL CENTER FOR SOLVING SPECIAL SOCIAL AND HEALTH PROBLEMS
169 Eleventh Street
San Francisco, California 94103
Phone: (415) 864-HELP

The National Center runs a Slim Chance program which applies Gestalt group therapy to the problem of weight control.

In Gestalt therapy, the emphasis is on self-knowledge. Members of the group explore their childhood attitudes toward food, their feelings about their weight and about losing it. Members conduct imaginary dialogues with their ideal self (the slender self) in order to understand their underlying feelings about their bodies.

The key idea is to Know Yourself Well.

Fees for individuals are five dollars. For group therapy, the rates run from twenty dollars to thirty dollars per month.

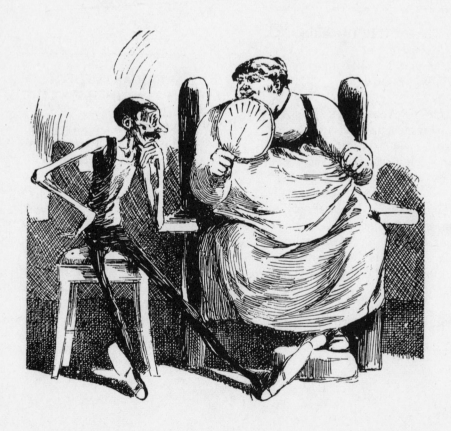

THE MILDRED JAMES METHOD
"Self-Improvement Through Relaxation"
Mildred H. James
P.O. Box 5203
Kent, Washington 98031
Phone: (206) 854-2461

Mildred H. James is a professional hypnotist who favors the group approach for weight control. Ms. James holds five-day weight-loss clinics through YWCAs and colleges throughout the West and Northwest.

The clinic format is one hour each day, Monday through Friday. The actual time under hypnosis in each session is thirty to forty minutes, with time for questions and answers before and after. The weight-loss course content is so structured as to enable systematic progression toward the goal of achieving complete relaxation, establishing new attitudes toward food and equipping the participant with the ability to use self-hypnosis. Cost is twenty-five dollars for members of King County YWCA; an additional four dollars is charged to nonmembers.

Cassette tapes are available for use as reinforcers by those who have attended Ms. James' clinics; or the tapes alone may be used by those who are unable to attend the clinics. They are available for fifteen dollars plus tax and mailing charges.

As my pal Willy Shakespeare once said, "To sleep, perchance to lose."

GOLDBERG'S DIET DIRECTORY

8 Feet of Listings

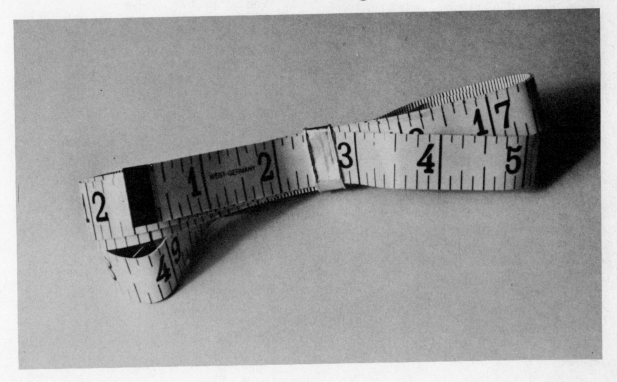

ATLANTA AREA CODE 404

Brown's Health Foods No 1. 3514 Fulton Av
  Hapeville
766-1767
Human Development Center. 5640 Peachtree
  Ind Blvd Chamblee
458-5882
National Diet Information Center. 1653 Execu-
  tive Park Dr N E
633-2241
Slender Wrap International. 6333 Roswell Rd
  N E
256-3107
Swiss Trim International. 5256 Memorial Dr
  Stone Mountain
292-6303
Weight Reduction Clinics Inc. 1874 Piedmont
  Rd N E
875-4733

BALTIMORE AREA CODE 301

Abbott's Health Farm Gambrills
987-0484
Riviera Health Spa. 6638 Security Blvd Wood-
  lawn
944-9177
The System. 6721 Reisterstown Rd.
358-7982
Universal Weight & Smoking Control Center.
  5602 Baltimore National Pke
788-4818
Weight Control Institute. 6615 Reisterstown Rd
358-8616
Weight & Tension Reducers, Inc. 6666 Security Blvd.
944-6060

BOSTON AREA CODE 617

Dance Theatre of Boston, Inc. Boston
423-9725
Dial Weight Control 15 Norwood Ave Newton
965-2181
Diet Workshop 100 Walter Roslindale
469-9254
Institute of Physical & Mental Development.
  1159 Hancock Street Quincy
472-4046
Schachter, Robert & Assoc. 1166 Beacon
  Brookline
738-0810
Weight Control. 15 Norwood Avenue Newton
899-5000
Weight Control Counselling Services. 424
  Newtonville Avenue Newton
965-4695

C C C C

CHICAGO AREA CODE 312

Ebony Reducing Salon. 221 E 79
873-7340
Edgebrook Bariatric Ltd. 6415 N. Caldwell
775-8787
Fruitful Yield Natural Food Store. 6606 Cermak Brwyn
788-9103
Garrett, Larry 6100 W Gunnison
774-9766
Goldsmith Drug Co. 3358 N Paulina
BI 8-5479
House of Nutrition Inc. 168 N State
782-3708
Hypnotism Institute of Chicago. 116 S. Michigan
FR 2-4188
Kramer's Health Food Shoppe. 29 E Adams
WA 2-0077
LBS Off Ltd Inc. 8324 S. Kilpatrick
585-2060
The Life Store. 1651 E. 87
731-2530
Management of Obesity. 7948 S Western
436-2552
NaturSlim. 4100 S Ashland
247-2990
Professional Weight Clinic Inc.
612 N. Michigan
266-0052
  Evergreen Park Plaza Evrgrn Pk
  499-3206
  2440 Lincoln Highway Olympia Fields
  481-1041
  685 W North Av Elmhurst
  833-5442
  3 S Prospect Park Ridge
  692-2683
  708 Church St Evanston
  328-3740
Professional Weight Control Clinic. 2739 W 55th
476-6262
Reducing and Weight Control Services
Academy of Hypnosis. 6100 W Gunnison
775-6100

Slim & Trim Figurama. 8142½ S. Kedze
737-3171
Slimjanes. 3000 W 59
471-1862
Trim Clubs Inc. 6677 NNW Hwy
775-6477
A World of Health & Specialty Foods. 2915 W Devon
274-9478

CINCINNATI AREA CODE 513

Clooney's Rosemary Aqua Slim Health Farm Inc. 8075 Reading Rd
761-2481
Diet Workshop. 7719 Reading Rd
761-7546
Figure Magic Figure Control Salons. 128 E 6
241-0507
  7610 Reading Rd
  761-1186
  3614 Springdale Rd
  385-3133
  6101 Glenway Av
  481-8444
  Cherry Grove Plaza
  752-7100
  485 East Kemper Rd
  671-0260
  Milford Shopping Center
  831-9742
Gloria Marshall Figure Control Salons
7292 Kenwood Road
793-6541
  Northgate Mall Shopping Center
  385-1600
  Tri-County Shopping Center
  671-6970
  Beechmont Mall Shopping Center
  232-1800
  2296 Alexandra Pke Southgate
  441-7536
Slend-O-Form Studio. 18 East 4th St.
621-3878

CLEVELAND AREA CODE 216

Conway Diet Inst. 23647 Woodhill Dr.
826-3479
The Diet Workshop. 13910 Cedar
371-9950; 371-2122

DENVER AREA CODE 303
American Clinic Inc. 1660 S Albion
758-4544
Anderson Edward G. 158 Fillmore
388-2411
Bernie Professional Building. 4950 S Holly;
2551 York
321-8473
Creative Concepts. Hiwan Village Evergreen
674-0234
Downs Linwood E. 1592 Madison
355-9048; 355-8911

DETROIT AREA CODE 313
Coprin-Community Professional Resources Institute Inc. 24901 Northwestern Highway
Southfield
353-4990
International Diet Centres Windsor Ontario
963-3438
Roseville Clinic. 31511 Gratiot Roseville
293-1100
Weight Watchers Inc. 318 Fisher Bg
872-2900

DISTRICT OF COLUMBIA AREA CODE 202
Diet Workshop of Washington, Inc. 8522 Milford Av Silver Spring
588-2330; 587-3438
Hilton-Stauffer Reducing Salons. 1215 Conn
Av NW
638-0453
Van Hooser Dr. F. L. 13000 Greenoble Dr
Wheaton
WH 6-7921
Weight Control Institute. 11141 Georgia Av
Wheaton
942-7900

FORT WORTH/HOUSTON AREA CODE 713
American Weight Control. 5322 W Bellfort
721-4792
De Jean Gene. 4007 Bellaire Blvd
668-5364
Get Slim. 1415 Hurley
924-8441
Get Trim Co. 6515-A Corporate
772-3687
Grace System The. 3917 Kirby Dr.
528-4390
Medical Slenderizing. 2135 Westheimer
522-2424
Medical Slenderizing Inc. 6565 DeMoss
777-8103
Shaklee Distributor. 3209 Ryan Av
926-5087
Slender Ade Inc. 2120 Ridgmar Blvd
731-3739
Slenderbolic Building and World Headquarters. 8320 Gulf Freeway.
644-2336
Trimlines Reducing Salon 1611 New York
275-3533
Texas College of Natural Health Sciences.
7021 Main
666-7112

KANSAS CITY AREA CODE 816
Alsop Diet Center. 6202 E. 12
483-5844
Get Slim International Inc. 1230 W. 67 Terrace
333-2080
Medical Weight Control Clinic. 667 S 55
287-1414
Professional Reducing Centers of America Inc.
1123 N 5
321-3204
Scientific Slenderizing Inc. 1000 W 47 Pl
831-0933
Slim-N-Trim Club. 3922 N E Couteau Trfwy
454-1559
Weight Control Clinic. 25 E 12 Street-Suite
814, 12th & Walnut St Bldg
12th & Walnut St Bldg
842-2337

KANSAS CITY AREA CODE 913
Professional Reducing Centers of America Inc.
Ranchmart Shopping Center
381-8131
6228 Nieman Rd
268-7000
Professional Weight Control Ltd. 11055 Cedar
Parkway
341-6161
Woodhead Diet Clinics Inc. 2210 W. 75th St.
262-2800

LOS ANGELES AREA CODE 213
Allen Medical Group. 3322 W. Beverly Bl Mtb
722-4300
    11678 Ramona Bl Elmira
    443-1707
    1830 S San Gabriel Bl San Gabriel
    288-3741
Alphagenic Psychological Associates. 7080
Hollywood.
466-3677
Ashton Health Institute Wilshire. 630 S Wilton
Pl
387-8953
Babcock Myron F. 1127 Wilshire
481-1750
Bruce Conner-Al Hinds Health Club. 10830
Santa Monica W LA
474-0029
Canoga Family Medical Group. 7110 Remmet
Canoga Park
883-8373
Cuilty Medical Clinic Inc. 1840 S San Gabriel
Bl San Gabriel
283-5554
Curry-Allen D DO. 127 W 7th Laguna Beach
775-1631
Dobson D. R. Hypnotist. 10922 Riverside Dr
North Hollywood
985-2012
Etienne Kathryn Madame Ballet School. 6272
Yucca
464-1794
Figueroa Health Group. 4601 S. Figueroa
233-4155
GMFC Inc. 9132 E. Stonewood Downey
771-1172
H C G Reduction. Dan W. Green MD. 2280
W Lomita Bl Lomita
326-1244
Hill Medical Group. 707 S Hill
623-4237
Imperial-South Vermont Medical Clinic. 11502
S Vermont.
756-1491
Inch Master. 3404 Cochran
931-7036
Inches-A-Way Salon. 5470 W Pico
933-8302

Julian Medical Clinic Inc. 2688 W Imperial
  Hwy Inglewood
754-2913
Karr Medical Group Inc. 7060 Hollywood
461-4668
  9615 Brighton Wyntoon
  274-9903
  3428 Motor Av Palms
  559-3277
  8215 Van Nuys Bl Panorama Cty
  988-7070
Keenan James.
556-3000
Kiowa Lodge Reducing & Health Resort.
  10633 Kinnard.
279-2332
Lake M Meredith. 6240 W Manchester
670-9200
Lead Response. 7712 Densmore Av Van Nuys
873-4900
Lee David Y. 4327 S Figueroa.
231-6745
Lindora Medical Clinic. 7080 Hollywood.
462-0883
  Hollywood
  462-0883
  Muir Medical Center
  Pasadena
  796-2614
  Crocker Bank Bldg.
  Hawthorne
  679-9236
  Hawthorne Medical Center
Little Bruce R. 10921 Wilshire Westwood
473-1146
Medical Weight Control. Downey 10250 S
  Lakewood
869-1477
  Inglewood. 543 W Manchester
  673-5800
  La Habra. 1881 W La Habra
  691-1223
  Van Nuys. 14349 Victory
  786-3702
  7304 Seville Huntington Park
  581-9566
Medical Weight Control Clinic. 12900 Venice
  Bl Mar Vista
391-6791

Mike's Weight Control and Non Smoking
681-6376
Mt. Washington Medical. 5224 N. Figueroa
255-1423
National Busibody Services. 6343 S. Eastern
  Bell Gardens
771-9666
Petersen Leonard E L 219 W. 6th
622-7209
Pioneer Medical Clinic. 1704 W Manchester Av
750-7965
Pounds & Inches Medical Reducing Clinics.
  5225 Wilshire
936-5233
Rust Harvey. 9060 Huntngtn Dr San Gabriel
286-7588
Schneider M. D. Inc. 5333 Sepulveda
390-4037
Simeon Weight Clinic Foundation. 6753 Holly-
  wood
464-7587
Soboba Medical Group. 9024 Burton Way
  Beverly Hills
273-0427
The Thinnery Company. 9337 Laurel Canyon
  Pacoma
875-3442
Thinnery The. 6280 W 3d
936-8877
Thin's Survival Food Program. 838 S Lucerne
  Bl.
389-2757
Tucker Jesse D C 3637 S La Brea
293-7838
Weiner Albert & Associates. 139 S Beverly Dr
  Beverly Hills
271-0361
Womens Weight Reduction Clinic. 6399 Wil-
  shire Bl
658-6700
World for Women Health Club & Spa. 3440
  Motor
838-7315
Zephyr Reducing Salon. 2607 Hyperion
661-3287

MIAMI AREA CODE 305

Dieters of America. 1921 NE 167 St. North
  Miami Beach
949-4747

Kennedy Clinic. 1900 79 St. Causeway
866-9044

Marcus Marilyn D O 18861 S Dixie Highway
253-0040

Medical Inc. 6781 SW 57 Ave Coral Gables
666-8573

  12316 W Dixie Hwy North Miami
  893-5586

NutriSlim Natural Weight Loss Program Distributor-Seibert & Webb Inc. 5855 SW 94 St.
661-0049

Thinweigh The. 6738 Pembroke Rd. Pembroke Pines
Miami Tel No 625-7335

Weight Control Medical Center. 11711 Biscayne Blvd
893-4480

York Health Products. 589 NW 62 St.
759-0711

MILWAUKEE AREA CODE 414

Diet Control Inc. 1723 Beech
762-4747

Perma-Slim Plan Inc. 5906 N Pt Wash Rd
962-6660

Persona Health Services Inc. 4709 W Lisbon Av
442-4141

Professional Hypnotherapeutic Services. 2457 N Mayfair Rd
453-2663

Rice's Deli & Legal Diet Food Emporium. 4610 W Burleigh
444-7060

Scotsland A Princess Resort. 1350 Royale Mile Rd Oconomowoc
Milw Tel No 342-0414

Seminars For Continuing Education. 1210B Sherman Evanston Ill. (312) 869-7345

Weight Losers International Inc. Exec Ofc 5500 W Capitol Dr
444-9100

NU YU Weight Losers. 5626 N 91
462-8370

MINNEAPOLIS AREA CODE 612

Seminars for Continuing Education. 2109B Sherman Evanston, Ill.
(312) 869-7345

Weight Away. 3944 W 49½ St.
926-2749

ST. PAUL AREA CODE 612

Alice Johnson's Stauffer System Salon. 1106 Grand Av.
227-6565

NEWARK AREA CODE 201

Birkett, Peter D M.D. 246 Clifton Av Clifton
843-2636
Diet Control Centers. 11 Stonybrook Rd W
    Caldwell
228-3729
Diet Control Centers. 1021 Stuyvesant Av
    Union
687-0007
Englewood Cliffs Milk Farm. 619 Palisades Ave
    Englewood Cliffs
568-5502
Essex Medical Weightcontrol Center. 15 Valley
    South Orange
763-0002
Hypnosis Associates. 246 Clifton Av Clifton
843-2636
Hypnosis Training & Consultation Center. 108
    Ridge Rd Suite 12 N Arlington
991-6083
Lean Line Inc. 1600 Park Av S Plainfield
757-7677

NEW YORK AND SUBURBS
Manhattan Area Code 212

Aesthetic Massotherapy. 90 Beekman
571-7979
Bertha Dingfelder. 20 Magaw Pl
568-6695
Browning Ed. 419 W 115
749-0307
Buonocore Frank J. 180 Thompson
254-9403
Cellulite Treatment Center. 16 E .79
879-8160
Dean's Reducing Studio Inc. 24 W. 57
265-9870
De Muccio Terry 212 E 83
249-2570
Diet Control Centers. 525 E. 88
535-9105
Diet Workshop The. 1975 Hempstead Turn-
    pike East Meadow
(516) 794-4881
Dieters Community Center Inc. 505 Park Ave-
    nue
421-1220
Englewood Cliffs Milk Farm. 619 Palisade Av
    Englewood Cliffs. N.J.
(201) 568-5502
French Richd 806 Lexington Avenue
752-6323
Galente Kenneth 102 E 66
879-4036
Gramercy Park Counseling Center. 38 Gra-
    mercy Park E
280-6001
Healthright Inc. 175 Fifth Ave
674-3660
Kahn Manya. 12 E. 68
BU 8-1300
Koytila Joe. 105 E. 37
679-0450
Peterson Penny 207 E. 37.
661-7780
Petrov Igor 1016 Lexington Avenue
TR 9-4676
Sam Victor 310 W 55
245-3136
Vitalla Slenderizing. 203 W 94
AC 2-4569

Weigh of Life. 430 W Merrick Rd Valley
  Stream Long Island
NYC Tel No 776-7812
Weight Control Dynamics Ltd. 171 W. 57
LT 1-9532
Weight Council Ltd. 30 E. 68.
879-8770

Bronx
Abbott Weight Control Center. 201 N Broad
  Phila Pa.
(215) LO 4-1022
Love Weight Watching Inc. 135 Dreiser Pl
671-2901
Reducing & Weight Control Svces 135 Einstn
  Pl
379-9578
Shape-Up Weight Control Center Inc. 1120
  Morris Park Av
931-1330

Brooklyn
Diet Control Center. 5 Snyder Ave.
469-3230
Hypnosis Weight Control Center. 2417 E 65
763-7614
Ideal Weight Ltd. 1701 Av M
258-0103
Lean Line of Brighton Inc. 2065 86
372-5844
Stauble Elmira. 3311 Church Av
BU 7-5733
Weigh-In, Ltd. 1616 Kings Highway
375-5315
Weigh of Life. 430 W Merrick Rd Valley
  Stream
NYC Tel No 776-7812
Why Weight Inc. 1424 Sheepshead Bay Rd
769-3737

Queens
A Queens Cnty Div of Counseling Svces. 172-
  33 Hillside Av Jamaica
739-3366
Diet Control Centers. 85-20 258 Floral Park
343-7068
Green Mountain. 230-10 64 Av. Bayside
224-6453

NaturSlim. 382 Forest Av Woodmere
(516) 569-0249
Trees Douglas. 119-49 Union Trnpke Forest
  Hls
544-6175
Weigh of Life. 430 W Merrick Rd Valley
  Stream L I
NYC Tel No. 776-7812
(516) 872-8181
Yuwan Co. 315 E. 48 Brooklyn
756-9043

Staten Island
Lean Line of Hudson County, Inc. 110 Roman
  Av
761-3525
Lean Line of S I, Inc. 548 Willow Rd W
761-4300

Nassau Area Code 516
Diet Control Centers. 85-20 258 Floral Park
New Hyde Park Tel No 328-8444
Diet Workshop, The. 1975 Hempstead Trnpk
  East Meadow
794-4881
Schiavelli Robert S. 606 Rose Blvd Baldwin
BA 3-6877
Seifert Hilde L. 39 Croydn New Hyde Park
GE 7-2659
Supervised Weight Control, Ltd. 175 Jericho
  Trnpk Syosset
364-1444
Think Thin, Inc. 11 W 3 Freeport
868-2731
Weigh of Life. 430 W Merrick Rd Valley
  Stream
872-8181
Weight Control Assocs. 10 Ely Ct. Elmont
285-6648
Weight Losers Club. 52 Randy Ln Plainview
681-8139

Suffolk County Area Code 516
Diet Control Centers. 27 Glenmore Av Brent-
  wood
231-4442
G & V Distributors Inc. 38 James Babylon
422-6868

PHILADELPHIA AREA CODE 215

American Institute of Hypnotherapy Counseling Center. 5918 N Broad
WA 7-0216
Better Living. 155 Bethlehem Pke
CH 2-6930
Budnick, Linda Rachael 2318 Afton
355-1671
Education for Living. 1714 Walnut
KI 5-6844
Parnes Joseph N. 1235 Pine.
PE 5-9381
Pounds & Inches Weight Reducing Centers Inc. 1737 Chestnut
LO 3-6655
Rocco, Frank. 9622 Bustleton Ave.
671-0569
Seltzer Jeanne Slenderite. 1218 Chestnut
MA 7-8900
Shape-Up Weight Control Center. Benjamin Franklin Hotel
WA 3-9166
Silva Mind Control. Bryn Mawr
LA 5-0720

PORTLAND AREA CODE 503

Body Wrap Inc The. 9415 NE Fourth Plain Rd. Vancouver Wa
Ptld Tel No 289-4028
Medical Diet Service Inc. 1544 SE Hawthorne Bv
233-5741
W L C Inc. 811 SW 6th
222-1666
Weight Loss Clinic. Medical Dental Bg
222-1647
   412 NE 120th
   256-1033
   3835 NE Hancock
   288-6577

ST. LOUIS AREA CODE 314

American Clinic of Hypnosis of Greater St. Louis. 111 S. Meramec
721-2600
Drake Institute of Hypnosis. 8421 Delmar
997-5510
Seminars for Continuing Education. 2109 B Sherman Evanston Il
(312) 869-7345

SAN DIEGO AREA CODE 714

Coronado Metabolic Clinic. 579 Orange Coronado
435-0164
Dray Alan. 588 3d Chula Vista
422-8311
Eat Yourself Slim Inc. 8701 Glenhaven
565-2511
Fashioned Figure Salons. 250 3d Chula Vista
426-2100
Gloria Marshall Figure Salons. 2860 Fletcher Plwy El Cajon
463-0269
   128 Fashion Valley
   296-0161
   2525 El Camino Real Carlsbad
   729-0914
   542 Broadway Chula Vista
   427-8163
Lindora Medical Clinic. 315 4th Chula Vista
420-9580
Luly Chiropractic Natural Hygiene Fasting Clinic. 4305 Ingraham Pacific Beach
274-2482
MD Associates Distributor. 3837 Bonita View Dr. Bonita
479-7704
Magic Weigh Figure Control Salon. 1762 Garnet.
273-1402
Rakow, Dick. 3938 Adams Av.
281-4586
Shape Shop. 4971A Clairemont Square Shopping Center
270-2071

Shiatsu Weight Reducing. 3960 4th
298-9757
Soboba Medical Group. 8312 Lake Murray La
   Mesa
461-1791
Stallion Oaks Resort. Ranch Boulder Creek
   Rd. Descanso
445-4179
Weight Reduction Medical Clinic. Clairemont.
   6070 Mount Alifan Dr.
292-9600
   La Mesa 6505 Alvarado Rd.
   582-3551
   Pt. Loma 3255 Wing
   224-2446
Western Institute-San Diego. 7522 Clairemont
   Mesa
292-4220
Williams Edward C. 7855 Ivanhoe Av La Jolla
459-2444

SAN FRANCISCO AREA CODE 415

Acupuncture-Sunset Medical Center. 2409
   19th Av
664-2250
American Clinic Incorporated. 1255 Post.
861-3552
American Weight Control. 655 Sutter
928-5888
Bariatric Medical Clinics. 212 Stockton
433-2333
Body & Mind Clinic
956-7546
Diet Workshop. 2533 Taraval
661-7200
Fat Liberation. Berkeley
548-2653
Ferriss Alfred W. 516 Sutter
433-1515
   2367 Ocean Av
   334-6345
Haskel P-DC. 1252 Bush
771-1243
Jarico Foods Bay Area Distribution. 1485 Bay-
   shore Bl
468-4810
Niblack Reducing Methods - House of Slenderizing. 220 Taraval
664-0074

Presant Herman M MD Inc. 1624 Franklin
   Oakland
832-4253
S F Slenderizing Center. 345 West Portal Av
665-6231
Santiago Robert. 133 Geary
956-7527
Slim Chance Program-FORT HELP. 169 11th
864-4357
Sunset Medical Center. 2409 19th Av
664-2248
Weight Reduction Medical Clinic. 2533 Ocean
   Av.
586-5757
Wein, George. 2200 Pacific Av
346-0675

SEATTLE AREA CODE 206

American Clinic Incorporated. 334 NE
   Northgate Wy
364-9221
Associates in Psychology.
Bellevue Office
454-2400
Evergreen Medical Group 11301-5th NE
365-3654
   12610 Des Moines Wy S
   243-5194
   800 Madison
   622-4816
Fenston, Jerrold J. 6535 Seaview NW
784-0500
Hypnosis Studio. 20125 108th SE Kent
854-2461; 255-2898
In Shape Fitness Center for Women. 6300
   Roosevelt Wy NE
524-6310
In-Trim Health Studio. 6423 Fauntleroy Wy
   SW
937-7026
Svoboda Marie Yoga Instruction. 1221 Queen
   Anne N
284-9536
Transactional Counseling Center. 911 E Columbia.
323-1661

LIST OF PUBLISHERS

Abelard-Schuman
  666 Fifth Avenue
  New York, N.Y. 10019
Ace Books
  A Division of Charter Communication
  1120 Avenue of the Americas
  New York, N.Y. 10036
Atheneum Publishers
  122 East 42 Street
  New York, N.Y. 10017
Award Books
  235 East 45 Street
  New York, N.Y. 10017
Ballantine Books
  201 East 50 Street
  New York, N.Y. 10022
Bantam Books
  666 Fifth Avenue
  New York, N.Y. 10019
Barnes & Noble Books
  Division of Harper & Row, Publishers
  10 East 53 Street
  New York, N.Y. 10022
Bookworks Books
  Random House
  201 East 50 Street
  New York, N.Y. 10022
Cornerstone Library
  Simon & Schuster, Inc.
  630 Fifth Avenue
  New York, N.Y. 10020
Crown Publishers, Inc.
  419 Park Avenue South
  New York, N.Y. 10016
Dell Publishing Co.
  One Dag Hammarskjold Plaza
  245 East 47 Street
  New York, N.Y. 10017
Dodd, Mead & Co.
  79 Madison Jvenue
  New York, N.Y. 10016
Dolphin Books (see Doubleday)
Doubleday Books
  245 Park Avenue
  New York, N.Y. 10017
Essandess Special Editions
  Simon & Schuster, Inc.
  630 Fifth Avenue
  New York, N.Y. 10020
Frederick Fell Publishers
  386 Park Avenue South
  New York, N.Y. 10016
Golden Press
  Western Publishing Co., Inc.
  1220 Mound Avenue
  Racine, Wisc. 53404
Grosset & Dunlap, Inc.
  51 Madison Avenue
  New York, N.Y. 10010

Harper & Row, Publishers
  10 East 53 Street
  New York, N.Y. 10022
Holt, Rinehart and Winston, Inc.
  383 Madison Avenue
  New York, N.Y. 10017
Houghton Mifflin
  1 Beacon Street
  Boston, Mass. 02107
Hunter Ministries
  1600 Townhurst
  Houston, Texas 77043
Mason/Charter Publishers
  384 Fifth Avenue
  New York, N.Y. 10018
William Morrow & Co.
  105 Madison Avenue
  New York, N.Y. 10016
W.W. Morton
  500 Fifth Avenue
  New York, N.Y. 10036
Nitty Gritty Productions
  P.O. Box 5457
  Concord, Calif. 94524
101 Productions
  834 Mission Street
  San Francisco, Calif. 94103
Penguin Books
  7110 Ambassador Road
  Baltimore, Md. 21207
Pinnacle Books
  275 Madison Avenue
  New York, N.Y. 10016
Pocket Books
  630 Fifth Avenue
  New York, N.Y. 10020
Popular Library
  600 Third Avenue
  New York, N.Y. 10016
Pyramid Books
  919 Third Avenue
  New York, N.Y. 10022
Random House
  201 East 50 Street
  New York, N.Y. 10022
San Francisco Book Co.
  681 Market Street, Room 244
  San Francisco, Calif. 94105
Charles Scribners
  597 Fifth Avenue
  New York, N.Y. 10017
Signet Books
  New American Library
  1301 Avenue of the Americas
  New York, N.Y. 10019
Spire Books
  Fleming H. Revell
  Old Tappan, N.J.
Lyle Stuart Books
  120 Enterprise Avenue
  Secaucus, N. J. 07094
Viking Compass Book
  Viking Press
  625 Madison Avenue
  New York, N.Y. 10022
Warner Books
  Warner Paperback Library
  75 Rockefeller Plaza
  New York, N.Y. 10020